BASICS OF PERFUSION & CARDIOPULMONARY BYPASS

Dr. GAUTAM SENGUPTA

Powered by
24by7Publishing.com

This book **'Basics of Perfusion & Cardiopulmonary Bypass'** by
Dr. Gautam Sengupta

All the printing & distribution processes of the book
is powered by

24by7 Publishing
13 New Road, Kolkata - 51, India
https://www.24by7Publishing.com
mail@24by7publishing.com
+91 9831 470 133
+91 9433 444 334

Copyright © 2025 by Dr. Gautam Sengupta
Cover Design by 24by7 Publishing
All rights reserved.

No part of this publication may be reproduced, transmitted, or stored in a retrieval system, in any form or by any means, electronic, mechanical, photocopying, recording, or otherwise, without the prior permission of the publisher.

This book is sold subject to the conditions that it shall not, by way of trade or otherwise, be lent, re-sold, hired out, or otherwise circulated without the publisher's prior consent in any form of binding or cover other than that in which it is published.

First Published in Jun, 2025
Version 1.00

ISBN: 978-81-984564-7-2

Powered by

24by7Publishing.com

ACKNOWLEDGEMENTS

I am greatly indebted to my teachers, the perfusionists, and the operating room OR technologists, during my training period. Observing them closely and taking note of their words on the subject helped me grasp the finer points of the subject.

A particular thanks to Mr. Uday Paramanik, who joined as a general duty assistant (GDA) and learned the tricks of the trade admirably all by himself, observing others. Those were the days when a Tullu pump, blocks of ice purchased from the market, extra lengths of tubing, and a bucket were used for hypothermia and temperature regulation during cardiopulmonary bypass. He adapted to the improvements and changes quite easily, cleared an approved course, and became the designated perfusionist of the unit. He walked all the way with me till retirement.

This write-up would not have been possible without the support of my family. My sons assisted with computer-related tasks and telephone communications with the publishing team. Their mother, a dedicated Obstetrician and Gynaecologist, generously took time out of her busy schedule to refine the language and ensure the text was meaningful.

The job of a perfusionist is multifactorial. Maintaining the fluid level in the cardiotomy reservoir, changing the perfusion mode according to circulatory demands, keeping abreast of the blood-gas parameters and making need-based changes, and timely communicating with the surgical team without raising concern are pragmatic tasks requiring tact.

PREFACE

At the very beginning of my career as a cardiothoracic and vascular surgeon, I was instructed to learn about perfusion and cardiopulmonary bypass. These were the early days and almost all the teams were climbing the steep learning curve of cardiac surgery. A comprehensive knowledge of the basics of cardiopulmonary bypass and the circulatory mechanisms goes a long way toward procedural simplicity and tackling emergency situations. I had many queries during the process of operating the heart-lung machine and had to witness procedural modifications along the journey. I had to figure out most of the answers for myself and adapt accordingly. This helped, not only in the performance as a surgeon, but also as the team leader.

The perfusionist is one of the key people in a team where a modification or interruption of circulation to vital organs is needed. The importance of the flow of oxygenated blood and the introduction of extracorporeal membrane oxygenation as a therapeutic tool have opened hitherto unknown territories for the perfusion technologist. Ultrafiltration techniques and new gas exchangers have enabled better maintenance of internal circulatory pathophysiology and tissue oxygenation. The perfusion technologists of recent times have to perform complex additional tasks with greater responsibility.

A Heart-lung machine designed by Dr. Saibal Gupta, and fabricated at a workshop in greater Calcutta, was built at an affordable price locally. There are records of success with this contraption, but for some unknown reason, the machine was not popularized.

The recent trend is towards information packed notes, which help in getting through examinations but diminish imaginative skills and the ability to read between the lines. I sincerely hope this write-up will help the young perfusionists and aspiring cardiothoracic surgeons in their quest for basic knowledge and understanding of cardiopulmonary bypass.

For Dreamers

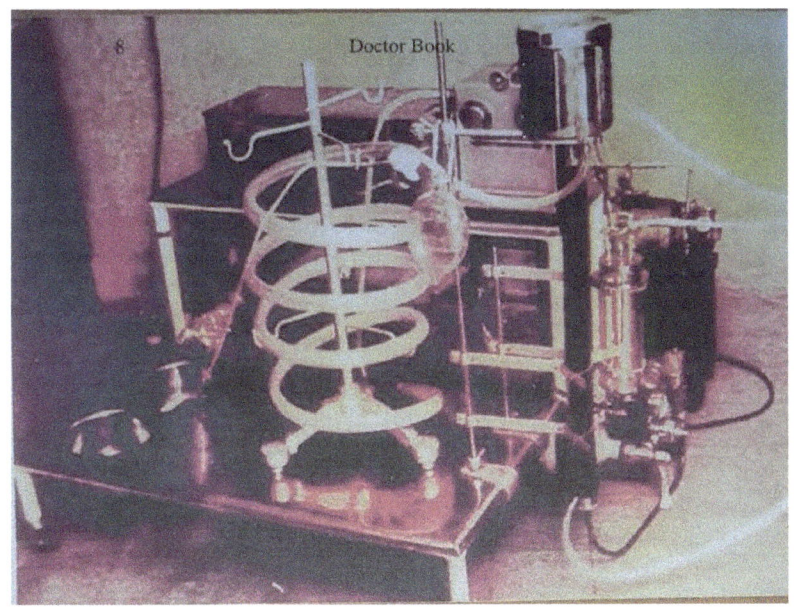

Calcutta Heart Lung Machine

Calcutta Heart Lung Machine 1962

First successful open heart surgery was done in August, 1962 using this indigenous Heart Lung Machine designed and made in Calcutta by Dr. Saibal Gupta, Research officer, Experimental Surgery Research Laboratory, at the Institute of Postgraduate Medical Education and Research under Prof. A. K. Basu, Head of Surgery. Surgical team was headed by Prof. A. K. Basu.

CONTENTS

Introduction 13

CHAPTER 1: Respiratory Mechanics 15
CHAPTER 2: Lung and Tissue Oxygenation 19
CHAPTER 3: Evolution of the Pump and Oxygenators 24
CHAPTER 4: DeWall and the March of Disposable, Collapsible, Polythene Oxygenators 31
CHAPTER 5: Membrane Oxygenators and the Hollow-Fiber Technology 37
CHAPTER 6: Additions and Accessories to Oxygenators and the Bypass Circuit 42
CHAPTER 7: Tubing, Flows, Cannulas and Connectors Used for Cardiopulmonary Bypass 48
CHAPTER 8: The Pump 56
CHAPTER 9: The Prime 67
CHAPTER 10: Adequacy of perfusion 73
CHAPTER 11: Cardiopulmonary Bypass—Procedural Details 76
CHAPTER 12: Recent Ideas and Additional Technological Applications 84
CHAPTER 13: Monitoring During Cardiopulmonary Bypass ... 87
CHAPTER 14: Gasses Used in Cardiopulmonary Bypass 95
CHAPTER 15: Cardiopulmonary Bypass in the Pediatric Patient 97
CHAPTER 16: Thermoregulation 103
CHAPTER 17: Anticoagulation in Cardiopulmonary Bypass and its Reversal 109
CHAPTER 18: Arterial Blood Gas and the Perfusionist 118

CHAPTER 19: Troubleshooting 122
CHAPTER 20: Conclusion 131

References *133*
Books consulted *135*
List of figures *136*
Index 138

INTRODUCTION

Cardiac surgery is relatively new, and only in 1896, doctors learned that tissue making up the heart can be sutured like any other tissue when injured and can function as before with little loss of contractile power. Before the feat of Ludwig Rehn of Germany, nobody could think of doing any surgical maneuver on the heart and the most influential surgeon of the time, Billroth, strongly endorsed this view. The heart and circulation are somewhat special in being dynamic always and all the operations have to be performed with the heart in a beating state and with the expectation of near-normal normal recovery. There was indeed a dearth of people who dared to handle the heart in injury situations surgically. Corrective surgery or palliation was never conceived and patients were left to die in such cases. Rehn's observations opened a new era and reports of success with surgical repair of heart wounds gradually filtered through. Thereafter, a few visionary people suggested corrective procedures for some conditions, but the actual procedure was performed successfully years later. The Trendelenburg procedure is a classical example. Though Trendelenburg proposed, operative success eluded him and in 1924, one of his students, Kirchner, succeeded in saving a victim.

From the early times, it was recognized that a contraption was required for some time to take over the function of the heart and lungs so that circulation, bleeding in the operative field, and oxygenation of the circulating blood could be controlled. The heart-lung machine, as it is called from the very first day, has a mechanism for propelling blood and into it is integrated a contraption for oxidation of returning and collected blood - the cardiotomy reservoir-oxygenator complex. Blood had to be collected and propagated through this arrangement in such a manner that there is no contamination of blood with the exterior at all.

CHAPTER-1
RESPIRATORY MECHANICS

For a better understanding of pulmonary gas exchange and oxygenation of the blood, respiratory mechanics have to be understood. Both lungs consist of about 480 million alveoli. The endothelium of the alveolus, which is the terminal air-filled dilation of lung tissue, is where the actual gas exchange occurs. 90% of the alveolar tissue surrounded by single-celled capillary endothelium is made up of flat type I pneumocytes. Diffusion is the process by which gas exchange between the external atmospheric air and capillary blood occurs across these pneumocyte-lined air sacs (alveoli). The alveolar membrane, where the actual gas exchange occurs, is made up of the flat type I pneumocytes, the capillary endothelial lining, and a thin basement membrane in between. The thinnest portion measures 20 nm. This membrane allows selective diffusion of gases without allowing virulent organisms to flow. The rest of the lung tissue is dynamically responsible for maintaining the lung architecture, form, and surface tension properties.

The pulmonary volumes and capacities are important for assessing the perfusion needs of an individual. The total lung volume/capacity is about 4-6 liters. In the living subject, the lung is never empty and an understanding of the volume and capacity subdivisions is necessary. The **tidal volume** which represents the usual amount of atmospheric air that is involved in the gas exchange during the inspiratory and expiratory excursions, is about 500 ml in the average adult individual. Next comes the reserve capacities -- the **inspiratory** and **expiratory reserve capacities** where a conscious effort is made at the inspiratory and expiratory phases inclusive of the tidal excursion. The **residual volume (RV)** is the amount of air that is left after the expiratory reserve volume is exhaled. The residual volume is the only lung volume that cannot be measured directly because it is impossible to completely empty the lung of air. This volume can only be calculated.

Lung capacities are measurements of two or more volumes. The **vital capacity (VC)** measures the maximum amount of air that can be exhaled during one respiratory cycle. It is the sum of the expiratory reserve volume, tidal volume, and inspiratory reserve volume. The **inspiratory capacity (IC)** is the amount of air that can be inhaled after the end of a normal expiration. It is, therefore, the sum of the tidal volume and inspiratory reserve volume. The **functional residual capacity (FRC)** includes the expiratory reserve volume and the residual volume. Lastly, the **total lung capacity (TLC)** is a measurement of the total amount of air that the lung can hold. It is the sum of the residual volume, expiratory reserve volume, tidal volume, and inspiratory reserve volume.

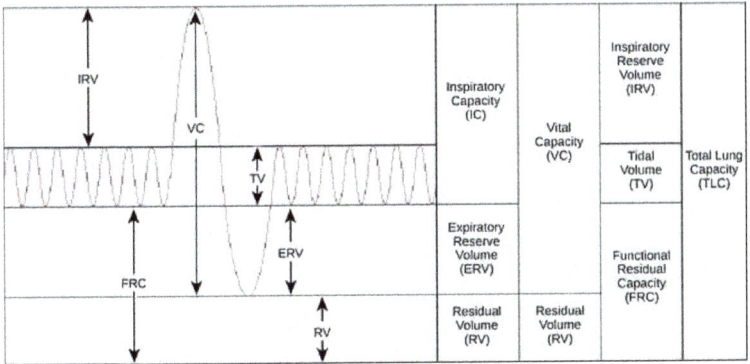

Figure-1. Lung volumes & capacities.

It is necessary to learn the value of the pressure exerted by the individual atmospheric gases taking part in respiration. At the very outset, one should understand that only oxygen and carbon dioxide are involved in the exchange, and the intricate interrelationship with the complex carbon dioxide metabolism has to be taken into account. Oxygen (O_2) is definitely smaller than the 3-atom carbon dioxide (CO_2), and once O_2 is adsorbed by hemoglobin, CO_2 cannot displace it.

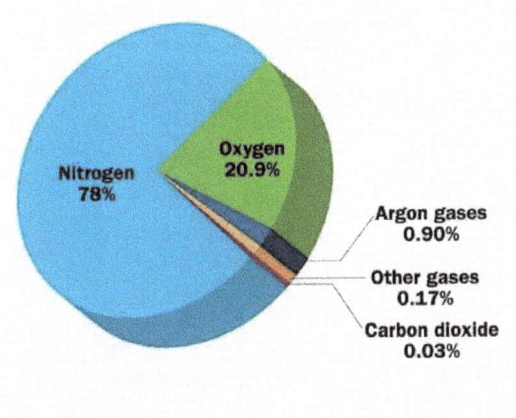

Figure-2. Components of air.

Respiration involves breathing in and out of atmospheric air. More O_2 is inspired and the expired air is rich in carbon dioxide. We know that the normal O_2 saturation in an adult is 95 to 100% in the atmospheric air. The atmospheric air is again composed of roughly 78% nitrogen (N_2) and 21% oxygen (O_2). The remaining 1% is a mix of mainly argon (0.9%), carbon dioxide (CO_2 - 0.1%), and other rare gases. Of this, only 2% of O_2 is dissolved in the plasma, and the rest 98% is absorbed for transport as oxyhemoglobin within the red blood cells after diffusion through a semipermeable respiratory membrane. To reach the cells, gaseous oxygen is liberated from both its bound oxyhemoglobin form in the RBCs and its soluble form in the plasma. It then passes through the interstitial fluid. Diffusion of CO_2 occurs in the reverse direction and is a combination of the following mechanisms discovered so far. After the utilization of oxygen in the cells with the production of energy for metabolic needs, CO_2 is liberated as waste.

CHAPTER - 2
LUNG & TISSUE OXYGENATION

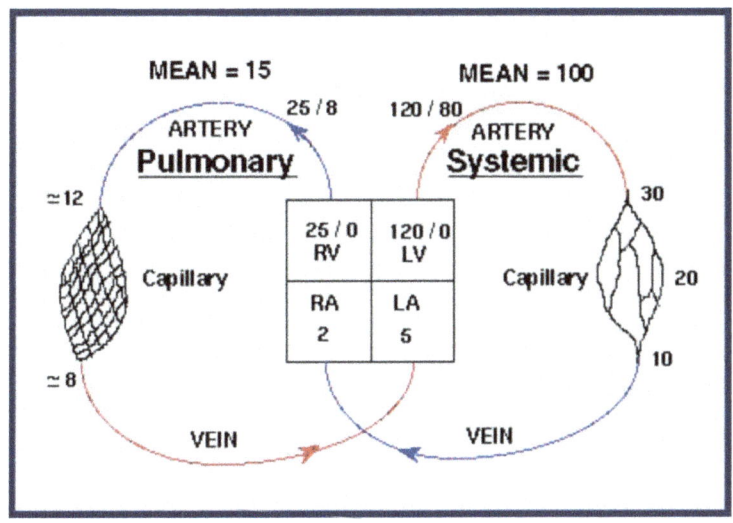

Figure-3. Cardiopulmonary pressures (cm of water)

A concept about the pulmonary vascular resistance (PVR) is important, that in simple words may be explained as, the force the flowing blood has to overcome during transit across the pulmonary circuit. It is measured as follows:

PVR = 80 x (MPAP – PCWP) / CO

(MPAP = Mean pulmonary airway pressure; PCWP = Pulmonary capillary wedge pressure; CO = Cardiac Output)

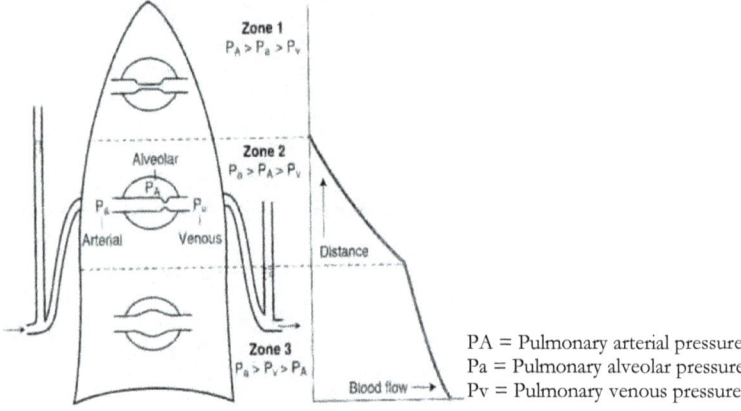

Fig. 4 'WEST' zones of the Lung & Pulmonary pressures

These are the 'West zones' and roughly demonstrate the relationship between the ventilation/perfusion (V/Q) ratio.

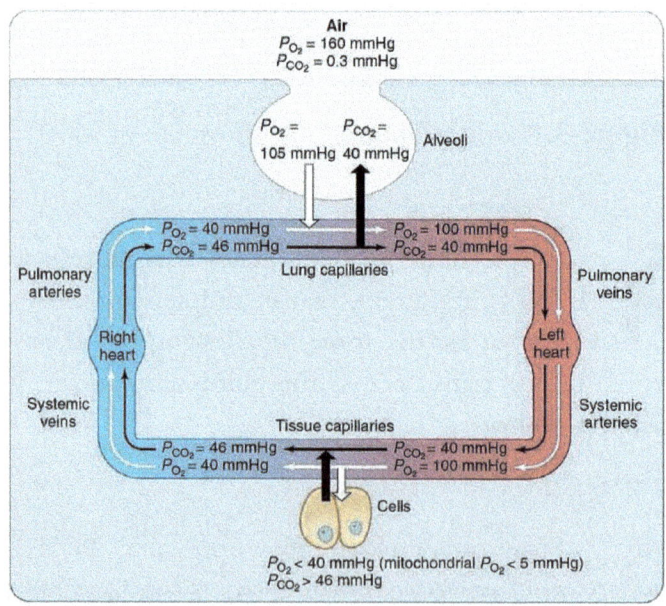

Figure-5. Oxygen and carbon dioxide exchange in the body.

The laws governing solubility of gases in a liquid and the principles ruling diffusion, and the laws of physics that describe the process of diffusion, are all followed during gas exchange. Partial pressure of O_2 and CO_2, pH, and the vascular resistances are important during cardiopulmonary bypass and perfusionists should have a basic knowledge of understanding cardiopulmonary bypass.

Inspired gas is diluted by vapor within the lung-tissue and reduces the partial pressure of oxygen. The partial pressure of vapor is 6.3 kPa/ 47mmHg and thus –

$$PO_2 = 0.21 \times (760-47) = 149 \text{ mmHg}$$

or

$$PO_2 = 0.21 \times (100-6.3) = 19.8 \text{ kPa (KiloPascals)}$$

The partial pressure of oxygen decreases again after the mixture of gas reaches the alveoli, where some oxygen is absorbed and CO_2 is excreted. The partial pressure at this point in the oxygen cascade can be determined by using the alveolar gas equation —

$$PaO_2 = PIO_2 - PaCO_2/RQ$$

The RQ stands for respiratory quotient and is normally 0.8. It is determined by the amount of CO_2 produced/oxygen consumed –

$$PaO_2 = 0.21 - 5/0.8 = 14\text{kPa } (106 \text{ mmHg})$$

O_2 transport or exchange across the membrane is simpler and adsorption to hemoglobin of the circulating red cells occurs.

A pressure gradient is always followed. Only 2% of O_2 is dissolved in circulating plasma and is inconsequential.

CO_2 partly is dissolved in the plasma (10%) and the majority (70%) is involved in HCO_3 production and in its assimilation. The enzyme carbonic anhydrase is needed for the creation and reversible maintenance of the ionic state –

$$H_2O + CO_2 \leftrightarrow H^+ + HCO_3^-$$

The part dissolved in the plasma directly diffuses out into the atmosphere across the barrier. HCO_3^- breaks into two parts -

1. A small portion slowly dissociates into CO_2 and water, with the gaseous CO_2 diffusing directly through the alveoli-capillary membrane (a slow path),

2. The rest enters the RBCs through designated pores instead of intracellular chloride.

   [This bi-directional movement of chloride ions in exchange for bicarbonates is also called the chloride shift. CO_2 liberated by the action of the enzyme carbonic anhydrase in the RBC freely diffuses out into the alveoli through the membrane. Thus HCO_3^- ions play an important role in maintaining the acid-base equilibrium in the body.]

3. The rest 10% of CO_2 is loosely bound with hemoglobin and the CO_2 is liberated into the alveolus in the gaseous form proportional to the partial pressures of O_2 and CO_2.

The intra-alveolar pressures at inspiratory and expiratory phases vary from a minimum of -1 to a maximum of +1 atmosphere.

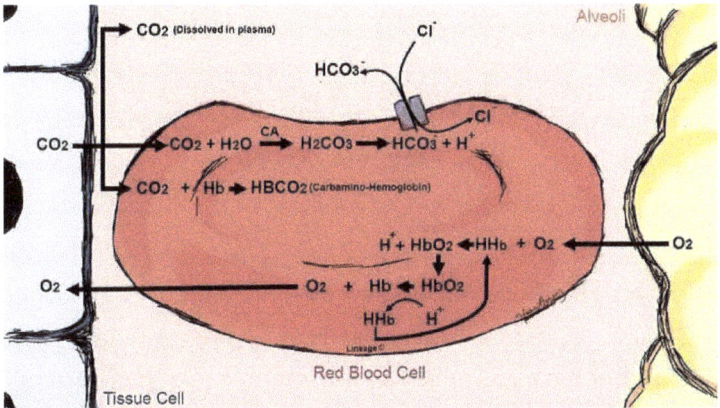

Figure-6. Oxygen & Carbon dioxide exchange pathways

This is a diagrammatic representation of the events that occur within the different environments. Between the capillary endothelium and tissue cells there is a layer of interstitial fluid that can be traversed by the smaller molecules in either direction facilitating the diffusion of gases. Gaseous CO_2 escapes into the alveolus maintaining an equilibrium with in-flow of O_2 in accordance with the cellular demand. A fine balance between the partial pressures of the two gases and the cyclical metabolic process in the lungs is always preserved.

CHAPTER - 3
EVOLUTION OF THE PUMP & OXYGENATORS

John Heysham Gibbon in his residency was entrusted with a patient diagnosed as being stricken with pulmonary embolism by his mentor, Dr. E. Churchill. Over the night he failed to do anything. He witnessed a painful death instead. This experience drove him to research a method for making safe heart surgery a reality under a controlled situation.

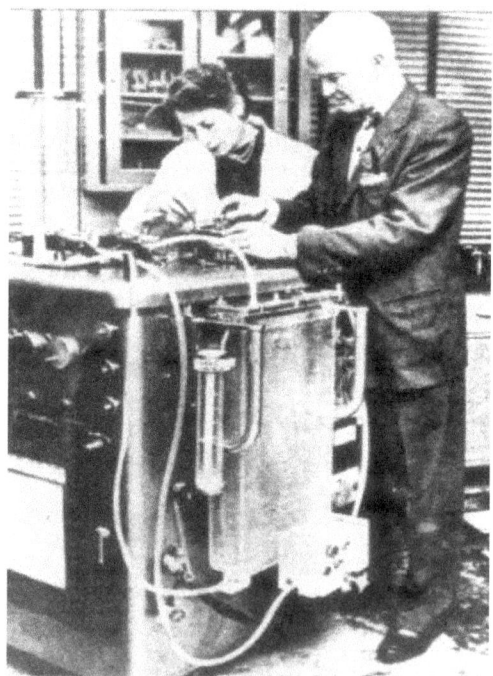

Figure-7. John & Mary Gibbon with their invention.

Initially, two streams evolved with the same basic principle of superseding and diverting the patient's circulation, either by the Gibbon-type heart-lung machine or, by connecting the patient's circulation to one of the parents with the same blood group, by tubing, in a manner that the parent's circulation takes up the burden of the patient's circulation. Thus, the patient's system could be isolated and surgery done in a leisurely fashion. This was Clarence Walton Lillehei's famous controlled cross-circulation method and he was able to do several innovative procedures.

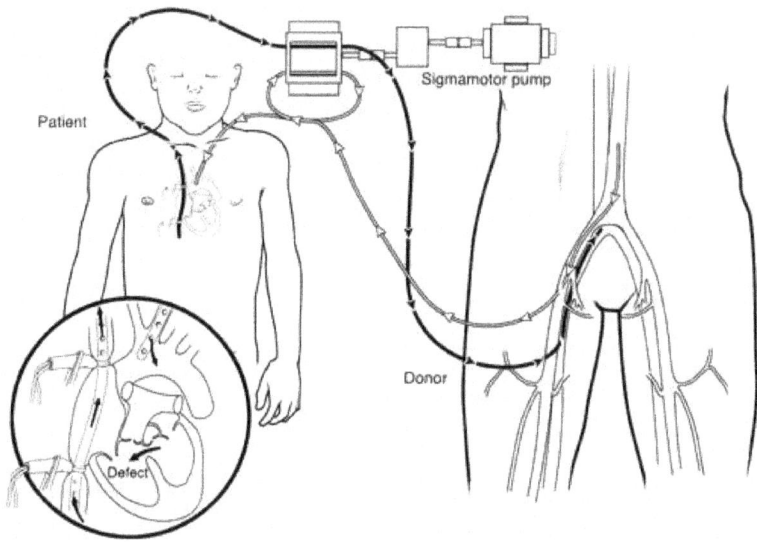

Figure-8 Controlled cross-circulation

According to DeWall, who was working with Lillehei at that time, a total of 45 patients with congenital heart defects were operated upon with the aid of controlled cross-circulation for one year from 1954 to 1955. Blood flow supplied to these patients was calculated to be 30% to 40% of the patient's resting output. The first patient, who survived, was a 13-

month-old child with a ventricular septal defect. The method had certain advantages—

1. Minimal blood priming was required,
2. Disposable heparinized accessories utilization could be minimized, and a simple connection between the donor and the patient could be ensured,
3. The scarcity of funds just after the World War II could thus be managed.

However, Lillehei's process had certain flaws, e.g.,—

1. The process endangered two lives. Thus, mortality had a 200% probability and encroached on ethical and moral issues,
2. Morbidity of the donor was a distinct possibility,
3. Operations could be done in low-weight and young patients only, lessening the burden of the parent's circulation.

Logically, Lillehei abandoned the cross-circulation soon and opted for the heart-lung machine.

A painstaking and methodical approach with a Gibbon-type heart-lung machine was carried on by Kirklin and his team at the Mayo Clinic in Rochester. Acceptable results made cardiac surgeons realize that utilization of the heart-lung machine was the way forward. Setting up of the contraption consisting of a pump for driving the circulation, a suitable receptacle for the collection of the venous blood and its defoamation with settling of macroscopic bubbles, and a membrane or a cylinder or a rotatable drum for oxygenation of the collected blood were needed.

The concept of oxygenation of blood to revitalize an animal that was failing was not new and in fact, Robert Hooke made this famous statement ---"I shall shortly further try, whether the suffering the Blood to circulate through a vessel, so as it may be openly exposed to fresh air, will not suffice for the life of an Animal; and make some other Experiments, which, I hope, will thoroughly discover the Genuine use of Respiration; and afterwards consider what benefit this may be to Mankind". This quote, Jules Verne-like, was futuristic at that time. To summarize, in 1813, Le Gallois theorized the first concept of an artificial circulation. "If one could substitute for the heart a kind of injection … of arterial blood, either natural or artificially made … one would succeed easily in maintaining alive indefinitely any part of the body." (Le Gallois 1812). In 1828, Kay showed that the contractility of muscle could be restored by perfusing with blood.

Le Gallois "oxygenated" the blood collected in a container by agitating it with air, to perform some gory experiments in the guillotined head of the corpses and highlighted the importance of blood in the perfusate solution to obtain neurologic activity in isolated mammalian heads.

Ludwig and Schmidt in 1868, built a device that could infuse blood under pressure, thus enabling better perfusion of isolated organs for study.

In 1882, Von Schroeder developed and built the first prototype of a primitive bubble "oxygenator", which consisted of a chamber containing venous blood; the air was bubbled into the chamber and converted the venous blood to arterial blood.

In 1885, Von Frey and Gruber developed the actual artificial heart-lung system whereby the perfusate solution could be oxygenated without interrupting blood flow. This was quite an achievement and the model was based on the theory of 'direct contact' oxygenation of blood prevalent at that time. Mere bubbling of oxygen through a beaker containing venous blood led to an immediate change in the color from dark red to bright red. Agitating or shaking blood in a container having some air inside had the same effect. What actually happened was oxygen was adsorbed by the hemoglobin molecule, due to a greater affinity, and carbon dioxide was displaced. Film and bubble oxygenators were devised first as the 'direct contact' theory. This was time-tested, and reliable, and any change could merely be verified by a color change.

The screen and the rotating disc oxygenators were next to be developed. Both Kay-Cross and Dale-Shuster types of rotating cylinder oxygenators were used. The size of the discs in the original model of the Kay-Cross oxygenator approximated to 59 corrugated circular discs (to increase the area of surface available for oxygenation) and the size of such discs varied from 5" to 25". The Dale-Shuster model had the additional advantage of having an integrated heat exchanger and incorporated a kymograph for blood pressure measurement and a spirometer for pre-operative assessment of the probable volume of air in the lung.

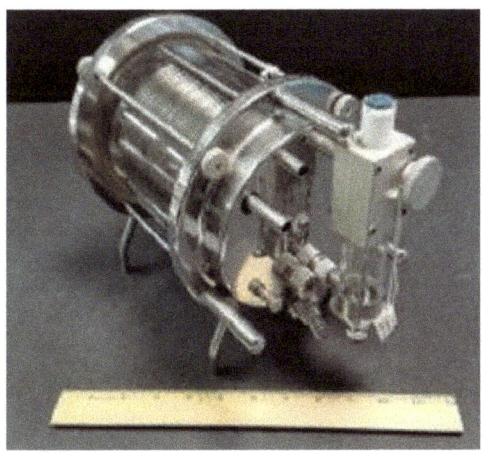

Fig - 9. Kay-Cross oxygenator

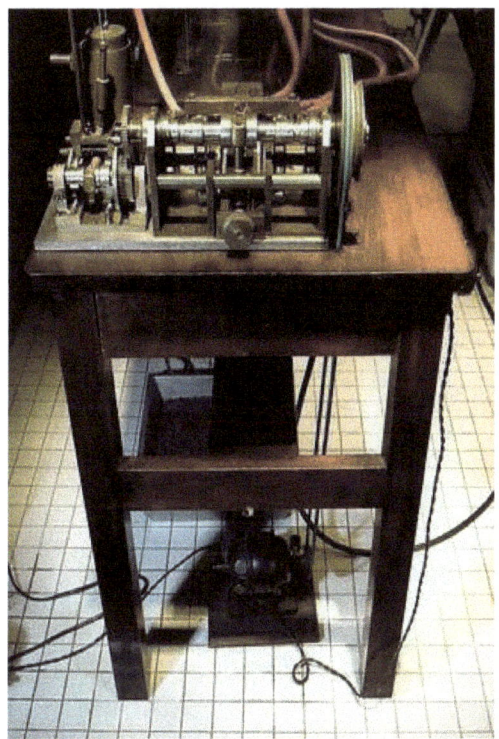

Fig 10. Dale-Shuster oxygenator

However, the cleaning and sterilization by autoclaving and the subsequent setting up of this sort of oxygenators with the pump in use, took almost the whole day. The process started early in the morning while actual incision on the patient was made in the late afternoon or evening hours.

There was also a vertical screen oxygenator on the same principle of direct oxygen contact. This had the advantage of feeding the anesthetic and respiratory gases into the oxygenator of the setup and was used at the Mayo Clinic, Rochester.

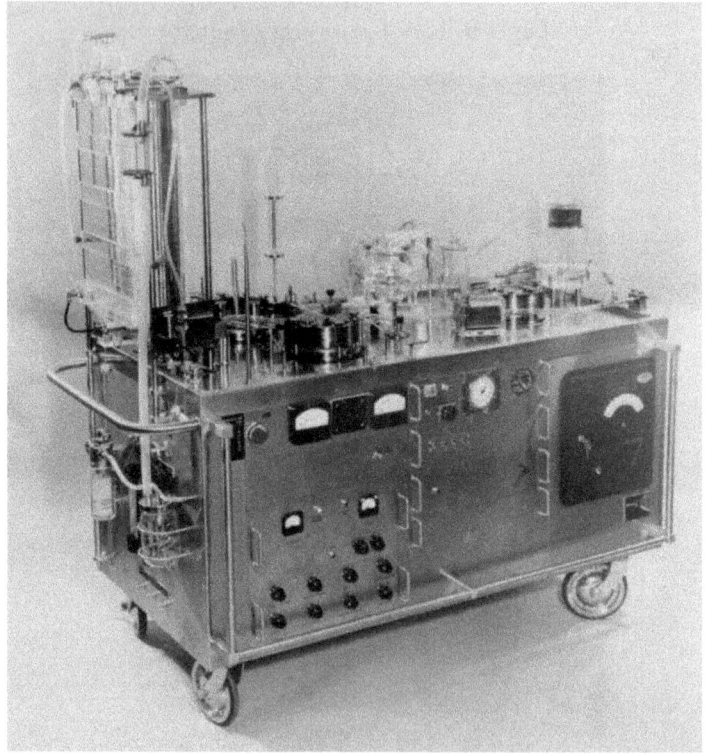

Fig - 11 Set-up for Cardiac surgery during the early days at the Mayo Clinic.

CHAPTER – 4
DEWALL AND THE MARCH OF DISPOSABLE, COLLAPSIBLE, POLYTHENE OXYGENATORS

Lillehei was doing cardiac surgery by the cross-circulation technique, developed by himself, at the University of Minnesota Medical School at Minneapolis. Lillehei performed open heart surgery after Gibbon had given up, and used the support of controlled cross-circulation as the unique technique in 1954. He visited the Mayo Clinic, where Kirklin was doing cardiac surgery methodically with a Gibbon type of machine integrated with an oxygenator and realized that this was the future. But the cumbersome nature of setting up the appliances did not appeal to him. Immediately on returning to his own unit, at the University of Minnesota Medical School at Minneapolis, he instructed Richard DeWall of his team to develop a simple bubble oxygenator where everything was housed in transparent plastic. Lillehei further suggested Dewall to look into industrial poly-vinyl-chloride (PVC) plastics as a transparent and flexible housing material. Though there were concerns, PVC plastics were inert, resistant to corrosion, and safe within the range of cardiac surgery.

It was realized very early that at least 1-4 m^2 of surface exposure was necessary for effective gas exchange for the construction of an oxygenator to act as the surrogate of lungs. DeWall soon came up with the first disposable plastic transparent bubble oxygenator that was first clinically used in 1955. Initially it could be used in patients weighing 20 lbs or less and appropriate age; proportionate increase in size with the ability for usage in adult patients took time. Though Lillehei was afraid of gas embolism and warned DeWall about bubbles, he allowed DeWall to proceed and as technology advanced, the bubble oxygenator device introduced by DeWall and Lillehei emerged as the safest and most cost-efficient disposable system worldwide. This particular oxygenator technology dominated the industry for 25 years and Cooley-Beall (1962) was the first commercially available bubble oxygenator. By this time several other investigators were in the fray and Gott's effort in producing the collapsible two sheet portable oxygenator is worth a mention.

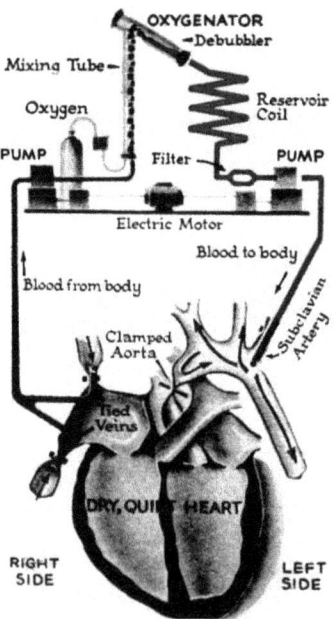

Fig 12 DeWall's oxygenator - scheme.

Several models of bubble oxygenators appeared in the market and gradually the hard shell polycarbonate resins, which were optically transparent, easily moldable, and impact-resistant oxygenators replaced the older soft and foldable models.

The ideal oxygenator should be as follows:

1. Safe.
2. Efficient in gas exchange.
3. Distance with the pump and the patient should not be a barrier.
4. Easy to assemble.
5. Risk of gas embolism should be minimal or nil.
6. Requirement of a small priming volume.
7. There should be the least trauma to blood cells.

If we consider the oxygenators developed so far then the following table is helpful:

Table-I

TYPES OF OXYGENATORS IN PRACTICE			
BUBBLE – DIRECT BUBBLING OF FLOWING O_2	FILM	MEMBRANE	LIQUID
	ROTATING DISC. FOAM. FILM OF BLOOD OVER SPONGE. STATIONARY SCREEN.	1. TRUE MEMBRANE. 2. HOLLOW FIBER. 3. NON-PLASMA PERMEABLE PMP 4. HOLLOW-FIBER MEMBRANE.	COMMERCIALLY NOT AVAILABLE

BUBBLE OXYGENATORS

The later oxygenators that depended on the 'direct contact' oxygenation hypothesis, added a "sparging plate" for regulating inflowing oxygen bubble size. This is a simple polycarbonate plate, perforated or with perforations sealed with porous silicate so that large oxygen bubbles are not formed during the inflow of the gas. Further, the de-bubbling and defoaming of the oxygenated blood occurred on entering the designated area inside the oxygenator filled with 175-micron polyurethane sponges, beads, shreds, meshes, and fabric threads. These are again coated with an antifoam layer of silicone. Bubbles are required for oxygenation. While larger bubbles lead to better washout of carbon dioxide (>25 times), small bubbles adsorb oxygen more efficiently. This is because of the different and comparative diffusion characteristics of these two respiratory gases.

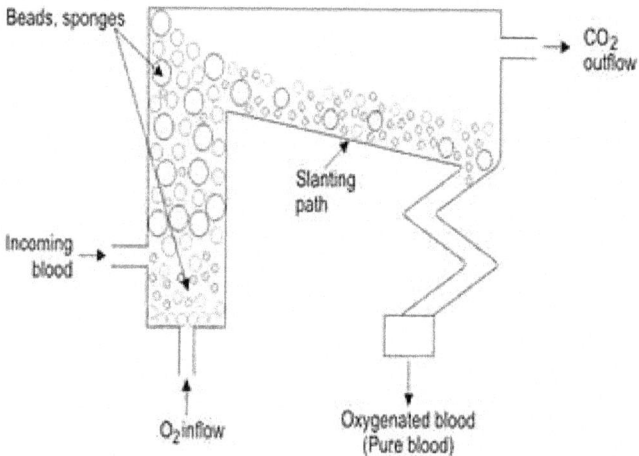

Figure-13. Principle of sequential de-bubbling in a bubble oxygenator

A compromise for efficient gas exchange is incorporated in the oxygenator and 3-7 mm bubbles are considered to be optimum. The blood, after the gas exchange, is decanted slowly along a slope and finally enters the arterial chamber ready to enter the body. Hence the later generation of bubble oxygenators were ready to assemble straight from the box, cheap, had good oxygenation capability, and needed a reduced priming volume. The inhaled anesthetic during the course of CPB is delivered via the membrane oxygenator, rather than the patient's lungs that are not ventilated during the procedure. Non-inhalational agents such as narcotics adequately supplement the inhaled anesthetic during the conduct of the operation. There were several companies in the market and Polystan was the only major soft, foldable, two sheet oxygenator available. Spictra was indigenous and Capiox, Terumo, Dideco, etc. were all imported and hard-shell polycarbonate products.

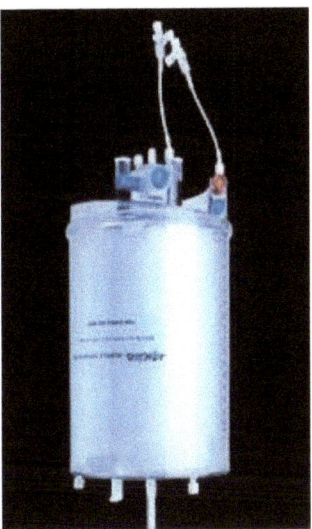

Figure 14. Spictra oxygenator

With time and with an intention for the development of safer oxygenators, the research continued. Gibbon's feat was done with a bulky screen oxygenator and initially the Mayo Clinic in Rochester, where Kirklin and his team resumed cardiac surgery, followed in his footsteps.

CHAPTER - 5
MEMBRANE OXYGENATORS & THE HOLLOW-FIBRE TECHNOLOGY

Membranes were explored next. The search for a less traumatic and more physiological oxygenating interface was inevitable as the bubble oxygenators, though highly successful in heart surgery and other procedures needing oxygenation during surgery, could work efficiently for only a specific period of time (4-6 hrs). Though oxygenation is very good with the introduction of gas bubbles, there are certain disadvantages --

1. Trauma to blood cells,
2. Coagulopathy,
3. Protein denaturation and capillary leak,
4. Formation of micro-aggregates and micro-debris
5. A potentially threatening whole-body inflammation with complement activation.
6. Higher probability of infection as gas bubbles get into direct contact with blood,
7. Chance of air embolism.

In addition, there was exponential development of extracorporeal life support (ECLS) and similar life-saving systems. These necessitated the development of a less traumatizing oxygenator that was only selectively permeable to gases and at the same time formed a barrier between the blood and injected gases.

Kolf and Berg in 1944 first noticed that the blood was getting oxygenated when oxygen-containing dialyser fluid was circulated through their dialyser machine separating the two fluids by a selectively permeable cellophane membrane. The potential advantage was immediately understood and a search was instituted for a quick and selectively permeable membrane allowing gas exchange and keeping the other constituents of blood unchanged. The membranous material had to be biologically acceptable to the body as well. Initially, ethylcellulose and polyethylene were found and soon replaced by the stronger polytetrafluoroethylene (PTFE) membranes or Teflon. In the beginning, the biocompatible membranes were stacked as a sandwich with a manifold in-between. Experiments with "arranged hydrophilic membranes" thus revealed internal leakage of plasma and had the problem of collection of blood which ran out of the oxygenator like thick rivulets. Hydrophobic isomers were tried next, but as Melrose, in 1958, pointed out that, though oxygenation was not a problem, CO_2 removal was an issue. All these reduced the duration for safe use. The creation and use of silicone as a diffusible membrane solved the gas exchange problem and the difficulties inherent to silicone (the "sticky mess") were tackled by forming a double-layered membrane with the scaffolding of a nylon net in-between the two layers. Continuous flow of blood created a selectively permeable biofilm which effectively occluded the pin-hole sized pores in the silicone membrane and thus helped to form a physical barrier between blood and gas.

Modern versions of silicone membrane oxygenators are still in use and are marketed as long-term extracorporeal oxygenators. Marks et al (1966) theorized that oxygen transfer into a blood film is proportional to the square of the thickness of the blood film and the diffusion resistance of the boundary layer. Further improvement consisted in creating thinner membranes and placing barriers in the path of blood so that eddy currents and turbulence are formed improving gas exchange. These are true silicone membrane oxygenators having a significantly long life, and are still used in ECMO and $ECCO_2R$ (removal) circuits.

Cardiac surgery needed highly efficient oxygenators where---

a). blood cells are minimally traumatized,

b). gas exchange is efficient, and there is

c). an effective barrier between flowing blood and the gas.

The Hollow Fiber technology replaced the true silicone membranes for greater performance within a limited time. This was an alternative process where extremely thin microporous hollow fibres made of polypropylene are used. The pore size was 0.02 nm and blood and plasma flow deposited a proteinaceous biofilm on the pores. This, along with condensed water created the effective barrier required to keep the blood and gas separate. Either could be inside or outside and the recent trend has been to design an oxygenator with blood circulating the outer aspect of the oxygenators. This is in variance with earlier and conventional "blood inside" devices and has been found to help in two ways:-

1. better gas exchange,
2. minimizes resistance to the flow of blood.

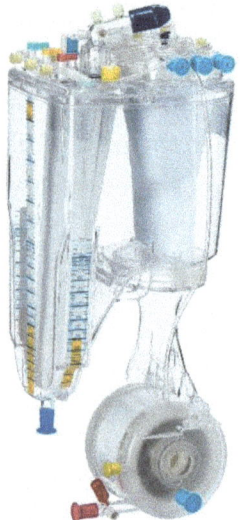 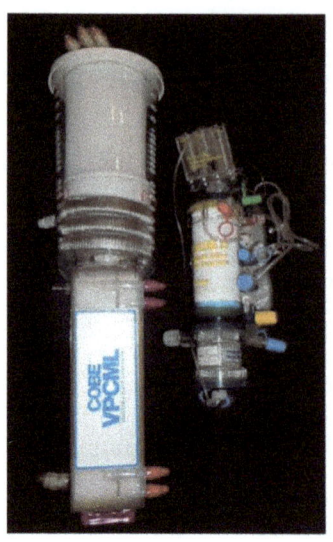

Figure-15a. An adult oxygenator.

Figure-15b. Both Pediatric & neonatal versions.

A successful artificial lung normally delivers about 250 cm³ (STP) per minute of oxygen and removes about 200 cm³ (STP) per minute of carbon dioxide.

In cardiopulmonary bypass, microporous polyolefin hollow-fiber membrane modules with a membrane area of 2–10 m² are generally used for gas exchange. An oxygenator can never replace the native lungs. With the use of an oxygenator, the goal is tissue circulatory delivery of 100% oxygenated blood with a $PaCO_2$ of not >45 mm of Hg and minimal hemolysis.

Oxygenator size can be --

1. Adult,
2. Small adult,

3. Pediatric, and
4. Infant.

Appropriate tubing size and length are used and the goal is to expose the patient's blood to the least foreign surface area.

CHAPTER – 6
ADDITIONS & ACCESSORIES TO OXYGENATORS & THE BYPASS CIRCUIT

The recent oxygenators not only had use in cardiac surgery (hollow fiber) or in extracorporeal membrane oxygenation and carbon dioxide removal (ECMO and $ECCO_2R$), but work was in progress with the development of intravenous oxygenation (IVOX) and implantable mini-oxygenators (IMO), having a hollow-fiber technology and low resistance to blood flow along the path.

The advent of efficient non-microporous hollow fibers made of new biomaterials such as poly-4 - methyl-1-pentene (PMP) is also promising. The material is almost as efficient as microporous hollow-fiber oxygenators. Non-microporous membranes are resistant to plasma leakage and increase longevity significantly. Thus, such materials have the potential to remove the hollow fiber oxygenator in the future.

True membranes have been used in prolonged extracorporeal life support systems when recovery is expected or during the waiting period for a donor heart in the 'bridge to transplant' period. However, analysis of retrospective and prospective data indicates that polymethylpentene (PMP) is used most and pediatric oxygenators have seen the maximum advances and they are empirically coated with heparin or the lipophobic phosphorylcholine. These PMP membranes can be used for a couple of weeks and will require a change when:--

- ΔP or pressure drop across the oxygenator is high,
- D-dimer level is rising with concomitant decrease in fibrinogen levels, and,
- Blood-gas analysis indicates sudden low PaO_2 with high $PaCO_2$ levels.

The COVID pandemic had a shattering effect on healthcare delivery, This viral disease has been feared for virulence, and infectivity, but posed new challenges. Smart designing, miniaturization, and ease of connectivity to the pump and tubings were quickly developed. New units were coming up with extracorporeal life support as the prime consideration. The use of extracorporeal cardiopulmonary support with ECMO to give rest to a failing lung, in terminal or near terminal situations became frequent. Oxygenators were modified and miniaturized accordingly, both for long-term use and quick change.

Table - II Frequently used surface modifications for extracorporeal circuits

BRAND	MARKETING IDENTITY	CHEMISTRY
Bioline	Maquet	Immobilized polypeptide with covalently and ionically attached heparin
CBAS	Carmeda	End-point covalently attached heparin surface coating
Duraflo	Edwards Lifesciences	Ionic heparin-benzalkonium chloride surface coating
Physio	Sorin	Acrylic phosphorylcholine coating
TDMAC	Battelle	Cross-linked ionic heparin surface coating
Trillium	Medtronic	PEG chains with covalently linked heparin
X-Coating	Terumo (Cobe)	Poly-2-methoxyethyl acrylate (PMEA)

[Surface coating materials (SMA) are decided by the manufacturer and are believed to modify and augment the anticoagulant properties of the foreign surface to which the circulating blood is exposed. Clinical data are, however, lacking and beneficial results cannot be predicted.]

Table – III The characteristics of oxygenators in the pediatric age group

Oxygenator	Medos Hilite 800 LT/ 2400LT	Maquet Quadrox-ID Pediatric	Sorin Liliput 2/ EOS ECMO	Eurosets ECMO Newborn /Pediatric	Chalice Paragon PMP Neonatal/infant/pediatric
Priming volume (ml)	55/95	82	90/150	90/190	65/145/175
Gas swap surface area (m^2)	0.32/0.65	0.8	0.67/1.2	0.69/1.35	0.45/0.88/1.23
Maximal flow rate (l/min)	0.8/2.4	2.8	2.3/5.0	1.5/4.0	1.4/3.0/4.0
Hollow fiber material	PMP	PMP	PMP	PMP	PMP
Coating material *	Rheoparin (Albumin+Heparin)	Bioline (Albumin+Heparin)	Phosphorylcholine	Phosphorylcholine	Rheopak (Albumin+Heparin)

(*Rheoparin, Bioline, Rheopak, and Phosphorylcholine are all surface-active hydrophilic agents, covalently bonded with heparin, which swell up on contact with the flowing blood and leave no chance for microclot formation. Coating the reservoir, oxygenator, tubings, etc., provides a relatively smooth contact surface, reduces chances of embolic episodes, and lessens inflammation in operations under cardiopulmonary bypass. The PMEA material has also been claimed to prevent platelet activation, clumping, and surface adherence to prevent microscopic clot formation)

ACCESSORIES

FILTERS

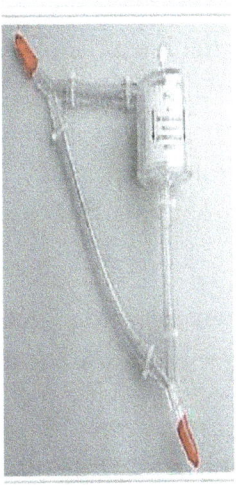

Fig - 16 Arterial filter

Filters in the cardiopulmonary circuit are essential and have to be deployed strategically to ensure adequate oxygenation before minimally traumatized blood enters the circuit. Prior to the final addition to the CPB circuit 0.2-micron filters in the gas inflow lines are always used to prevent bacterial or particulate contamination. Similarly, all crystalloid priming and cardioplegia solutions are passed through 0.2-micron filters. These effectively remove organisms like bacteria. One has to remember here that the diameter of the discoid red cell containing hemoglobin ranges from 7 to 7.5 microns and the maximal diameter of the largest blood cell, or the monocyte, is about 15-18 microns. It is obvious that placing a filter will require an extra driving force necessary to overcome the additional resistance created.

Consequently, trauma to blood cells will be greater. However, a non-resistant, primed, and adequately de-aired arterial filter is normally placed at the path of the arterial line to prevent any micro-aggregates, debris, micro-bubbles, and micro-clots from entering the arterial line to the body. The arterial filter is essential as it also is able to catch the 'spalling' debris created in a roller pump after prolonged use when the dumblehead of the roller repeatedly brushes against the siliconized PVC tubing lying static with a stainless-steel board behind.

The dedicated oxygenators for small babies and the prolonged life support systems use the integrated arterial line filtration (IALF) system.

The potential of a liquid membrane with liquid fluorocarbons is exciting. This has been found to reduce hemolytic damage and facilitate gas exchange. Though studies have been going on since the early '70s, a commercially viable model is still not available.

GAS BLENDERS

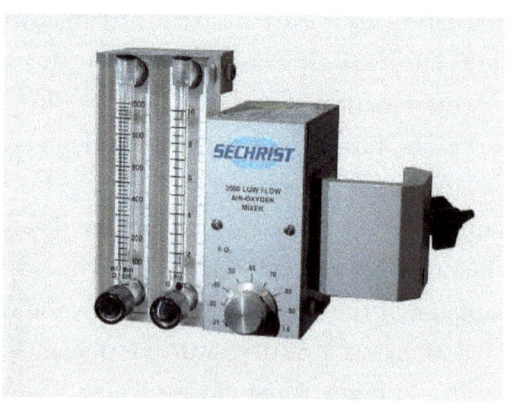

Fig 17 Gas blender

Actually, two such blenders become necessary for an operation of the heart under cardiopulmonary bypass. One is dedicated and fixed with the anesthesia machine, while the other is mounted to the heart-lung machine for delivery of oxygen or compressed air to the oxygenator.

CHAPTER – 7
TUBINGS, FLOWS, CANNULAS & CONNECTORS USED FOR CARDIOPULMONARY BYPASS

TUBINGS & FLOWS

Some of the most common types of plastic tubing include:

- ABS or Acrylonitrile butadiene styrene.
- Ethyl Vinyl Acetate (EVA)
- Nylon (polyamide)
- Polycarbonate.
- Polyethylene (PE) [Low & High-Density Polyethylene (LDPE & HDPE)].
- Polypropylene (PP)
- Polyurethane (PU)
- Polyvinyl Chloride (PVC)

Tubes for water and gas transport can be of any material and commonly these are wire reinforced. Ideally, tubes that will be associated with the carriage of blood and compressed by rollers of the heart-lung machine should be biocompatible, pliable and durable, transparent, and leakproof. The internal surface should be smooth, minimally or non-thrombogenic, and allow passage of blood with the least resistance. Of late, PVC tubing are preferred and the inner wall has coatings of silicone as a defoaming agent and a lipophilic agent that lower platelet adherence, micro-clot formation, and bleeding tendencies.

Table-IV

TUBING INT. DIA. (in)	PRIMING VOLUME (ml/ft)	ARTERIAL FLOW (ml/min)	VENOUS RETURN (ml/min)
1/8	2.4	<450	250-300
3/16	5.4	<1300	500-650
1/4	9.6	<3000	1200-1600
3/8	21.6	>5000	4000-4500
1/2	38.4	To maintain an acceptable hemolysis, flow velocity should not be above 200 cm/sec	>4500 and approaching 7liters

A ½ inch tube is seldom used except, possible, in adults requiring exceptionally high flows. In actual practice, several events depend on eye estimation and on the basis of prior experience. Recent work involves the use of pre-cut tubing lengths, also called the 'custom packs', as this saves time and limits the distance beyond which the heart-lung machine with its accessories can be placed.

CANNULA FOR CARDIOPULMONARY BYPASS

The cannulae are either arterial or venous and are required for direct vascular access during cardiopulmonary bypass.

Usually, the venous cannulae are larger than their arterial counterparts as they are required to collect a large amount of central venous blood depending on siphoning alone (in roller pumps) or depending upon the negative force created once the impeller of a centrifugal pump starts to rotate. The end opening of a venous cannula is larger and there are additional holes near the tip. Wire reinforcement is necessary when a degree of rigidity is needed for secure placement to prevent collapse. A large, wide-bored, and wire reinforced cannula (to prevent kinking and compromised drainage) is directly introduced into the atrium and the tip is positioned in the inferior vena cava. This drains both the superior and inferior vena cava (SVC and IVC) sufficiently so as to both decompress the heart and maintain a safe level in the venous reservoir. This is done only in situations where an intracardiac shunt is not present and no manipulation of the right side of the heart is required. For adequate drainage the manufacturing units have developed strategies in designing different types of collecting ends unique to a company. Thus the cannula tips may be :--

- Lighthouse tip.
- Full lumen tip,
- Basket tip,
- Bullet tip,
- Pilot tip.

Wire reinforcement is occasionally necessary for prevention of accidental kinking with the tube in place. This drastically diminishes the venous return. The majority of the venous cannulae are circular in cross-section. The end outside the heart flares wider so that it can be connected to a 3/8 or a ½ inch tubing via a secure connector to the venous reservoir. Pacifico designed a curved metal tip cannula for direct insertion into the vena cavae, allowing extra space for the surgeon. Nowadays pre-formed right angled cannulae, with or without wire reinforcement or with non-detachable metal tips, are available.

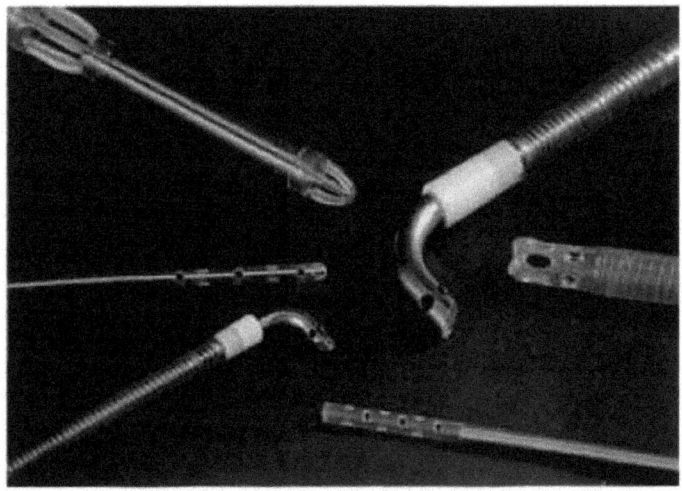

Fig -18 Introducing end of venous cannulas

Arterial cannulas are stiffer than their venous counterparts and these may or may not be wire reinforced. The portion entering the artery is beveled with a sharp edge and the end opening should look downward. The end-hole is always single and the probability of "sandblasting" the aortic wall where the arterial jet hits cannot be ruled out. There should always be a portion of the cannula within the aorta, and this should be palpated without fail for confirmation of position before applying the cross-clamp. Double, concentric, non-absorbable, purse-string sutures are taken in a circular fashion with suture ends protruding laterally, on the ascending aorta, a centimeter or so proximal to the origin of the brachiocephalic trunk. The suture ends are held together with soft rubber or plastic tubing fashioned from sectioned rubber catheters or disposable transfusion sets, and these are tightened in such a fashion that the snuggers lie just above and are fixed to protruding notched flanges or rings (single or concentric double) on the cannula just on the outside. Thereafter the arterial cannula spreads wider gradually to accommodate at ⅜ x ⅜ (in adults) or a ¼ x ⅜ (in small babies) connector for final air-free attachment with the arterial side of the heart-lung machine. Arterial cannula for cardiopulmonary bypass can be wire reinforced as well, and when not, should be malleable enough to be secured firmly with the least chance of kinking and obstruction to flow during bypass. Metal-tipped arterial cannula have the best internal diameter as these are strong and thin. Consequently, cannulation is easier.

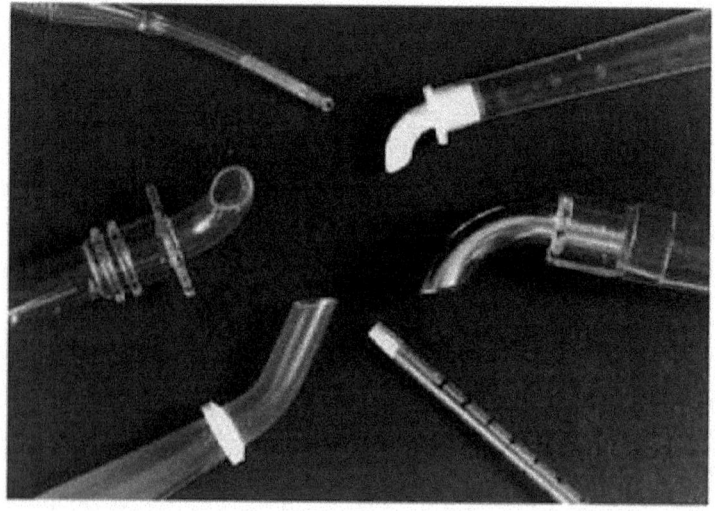

Fi -19 Examples of different types of arterial cannulas

BASICS OF PERFUSION & CARDIOPULMONARY BYPASS

The preferred sites for cannulation include the following:-

1. Arterial →

   a) Ascending aorta about $1\text{-}1\frac{1}{2}$ cm from the origin of brachiocephalic trunk – for central cannulation.

   b) Femoral artery – for peripheral cannulation and central cannulation in minimally invasive procedures, ECLS, and dire situations like cardiac injury during redo-sternotomy procedures.

   c) Axillary artery – for peripheral cannulation and MICS procedures.

   d) Brachiocephalic or innominate artery cannulation in proximal aortic dissection and arch procedures. This may be combined with a left common carotid cannulation and is a good route for antegrade cerebral protection in deep hypothermic cerebral arrest (DHCA).

2. Venous →

   a) SVC & IVC for individual single venous cannulae through the right atrium.

   b) Right angled cannulae of the SVC & IVC.

   The proximal part of the central veins are chosen and in most cases, a single purse string with snugged suture ends suffices. One should be careful of not injuring the SA node while cannulating the SVC for its proximity to the atrio-caval junction. A sufficient portion of the cannula should be inside the central veins to ensure adequate venous drainage. However, too large a portion of the cannula within the IVC is fraught with impeded hepatic venous return thereby decreasing total venous return as a whole.

c) Atrial cannulation through a right atrial appendage purse string in selected cases where the right side of the heart does not require to be opened and where an R-L shunt is not present.
d) Innominate vein, in special situations and in babies. The Innominate vein may be a good cannulation strategy for retrograde cerebral protection in DHCA situations.

Individual caval cannulation with snaring gives the operator extra space for intracardiac repair, especially in transatrial repairs.

Minimally invasive cardiac surgery has opened a new vista of ultrasound-guided percutaneous arterial and venous cannulations. A balloon at the tip and an end hole at the catheter tip positioned by ultrasound beyond the origin of the innominate artery from the ascending aorta solves both the problems of cross-clamp and antegrade root cardioplegia at one go. But the results of scrutiny in the matter showed unacceptable damage to the endothelial layers by the prolonged balloon pressure.

Ultrasound-guided transcutaneous venous cannulation technique is based on the modifications of the Seldinger method and Amplatz catheters are freely used for a gradual dilatation.

Ultrasound also helps in the positioning of these catheters. The Femoral vein and the right internal jugular vein are the usual access vessels when single-stage cannulae are used. However, a two stage cannula can be used and the point of entry is a single vein. Extracorporeal life support and minimally invasive cardiac surgery remain the most common applications.

CONNECTORS

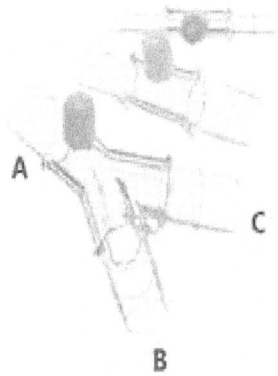

Fig - 20 Connectors

Of the other disposables in the cardiopulmonary bypass circuit mentionable were the connectors. These were biocompatible hard PVC material used to join cannulae and tubing in a leakproof manner. The connectors have non-return ridges so that such joints are not likely to give way during an operation in case there is an untoward rise in flow pressure at any one-time. In fact, the connecting region of the oxygenators, reservoirs, and filters, etc., are made the same way. These can be straight or Y-shaped and available as ¼", ⅜", and ½" sizes. The Luer lock on top or at one side is optional. When there is a size discrepancy, such as when a ½" tube end is to be connected to a ⅜" tube or vice versa, one side of the connector has a ½" joining end while the other has a ⅜" end. Similar reduction or augmentation of size is done with appropriately shaped and sized connectors. These are called 'reducers' in industrial parlance.

CHAPTER - 8
THE PUMP

The pump represents the heart in cardiopulmonary bypass and drives blood into the arterial system for circulating to the tissue of the organs. This pump is somewhat different from other industrial pumps -

a) These machines have to be forward-flowing kinetic pumps.
b) Leak-proof connectors for two ends have to be present,
c) There should be no contact of the fluids meant for the body with any external material, either within the pump or outside.

Actually, these move a column of blood enclosed either in a tube or a hard transparent polycarbonate shell. Examples are:

1. The roller pump
2. Piston-driven pumps
3. Finger or piano key pumps
4. Centrifugal pumps

The roller pumps were the earliest to be employed and commonly used, with a simple operating principle, and have been successful in cardiopulmonary bypass. The first roller pump was patented in 1855 by Porter and Bradley and was hand-operated. E.E. Allen, in 1887, made necessary modifications so that such pumps could be used for rapid blood transfusion when need. A retrospective search shows the next effort of medical utilization and modification of these roller pumps was by Michael DeBakey. He also found use for a smaller version of the pump with attached tubes and needles in rapid transfusion situations. DeBakey's paper (*A simple continuous-flow blood transfusion instrument* -- published at the 'New Orleans Medical and Surgical Journal' in 1934). The pump was electrically powered by Fleisch in 1935. By this time, Gibbon was exploring the hypothesis of isolating the heart and lung from the body during operation on the heart so that the field was not obscured. Animal (cat) experiments were underway and at this time DeBakey suggested the use of the modified roller pump as a substitute for the heart for maintaining a viable circulation during the operative period. In 1953, Gibbon made history by doing the first successful repair of an atrial septal defect in a young woman. The industrial giant IBM joined the race and J. Kirklin at the Mayo Clinic, Rochester, Minnesota, carried on systematically with the Gibbon-IBM type heart-lung machine with an incorporated screen oxygenator.

Before Gibbon's feat, (just before and during the early years after) the results were poor. Heart surgery involved mitral commissurotomy, PDA interruption, coarctation correction, and a handful of ASD closures, either by the inflow occlusion technique or the controversial Gross technique, well attempted at limited centers in America and Canada (specifically Toronto). Only 5 medical centers were actively involved in the development of the heart-lung machine. The early enthusiasts built a device on their own beliefs and attempted intracardiac repair with little experience and disastrous results. William Mustard at Toronto, Canada, even tried using a monkey lung with one improvised device in an attempt. Forrest Dodrill at the Wayne medical school in

Detroit enlisted the help of General Motors and built the Dodrill-GMR pump, which almost tasted success before the Gibbon-IBM feat. However, Gibbon failed in his next attempts and imposed a moratorium on himself awaiting validation from further laboratory results. It took Kirklin's disciplined approach and Lillehei's innovative brilliance to make open heart surgery a viable option.

Andreasen and Watson had shown before that the flow in the azygos vein to the heart was enough to sustain an organism for 30 minutes (article published in the *British Journal of Surgery* by A.T. Andreasen, and F. Watson, which reported the discovery of the "azygos flow principle," Andreasen JT, Watson F. Experimental cardiac surgery, 1952). Lillehei and his team used the adult human body, usually one of the parents with the same blood group, as a living alternative to the patient's heart-lung circulatory drive during the operative correction of numerous congenital cardiac defects. The patient had to be a child of the parent and have the same blood group. The heart of the parent had to sustain an extra circulatory load during the operative period. There were thus two patients, and the name '*controlled cross-circulation*' was given.

However, operations with a 'controlled cross-circulation' were only performed between 1954 and 1955. In 1955, Lillehei introduced the simplified and disposable DeWall helical bubble oxygenator. Operating with this oxygenator in place of a live patient was instrumental in the universal acceptance of cardiac surgery for all age and weight groups.

For the next few decades, further development occurred in the design of a better and more efficient roller pump only and these peristaltic pumps were found to perform satisfactorily and deliver adequate volumes needed for the maintenance of a circulatory requirement during the lower metabolic activity in hypothermic states. Hypothermia and different stages of hypothermia during operations, and the effect of low temperature on the outcome as the heart was in an arrested state for a period were extensively studied. Bigelow's name stands out as the principal contributor.

The roller pump used as the mechanical alternative heart during the operative period had minimal parts and a simple design --

1. The pump moved a column of blood/fluid by peristaltic massage,
2. The fluid had to be within a compressible tubing,
3. The compressive part of the roller for optimum effectivity in moving fluids is also known as the head. The roller pumps are categorized as single, double and multiple roller pumps. The single roller pumps were used for CPB in the middle of the 20th century. The flow in this type was more pulsatile. The most commonly used pump for CPB is the double-roller pump. This pump consists of a 210° semicircular support plate and two rollers with the rotating arms set 180° apart. When one roller ends its operational phase, the second roller has already begun its phase. Due to haemolysis issues, the third type (multiple roller pump) is not clinically available.
4. The rigid track (racing track) along which the tube is designed in a U-shape, with one compressive roller engaging the tube on the tract and the other disengaging,

5. Appropriately sized bushes hold the tube in place at the entry and exit regions, and the compressive rollers are also designated as the leading and trailing ones.
6. The occlusion should be strong enough to compress the tube and move a column of fluid within the tube uniformly along the length. Back-flow due to leakage causes more haemolysis and a total occlusion not only increases the haemolytic burden, but also raises the probability of causing a vacuum induced cavitation and small bubble formation inside the column of moving blood. Damage to the tube by 'spalling' is another issue where there is flaking of the inner lining if the compressive force by the roller is beyond optimum.
7. There may be two tracks with respective appropriately sized bushes in a pump. Normally the heart lung machine contains 4-5 roller pump units arranged side-to-side.

There are three materials currently used for tubing in the medical device industry: silicone, latex, and polyvinyl chloride (PVC). Regarding micro-particle release, PVC performs best.

Latex is more haemolytic and silicone tubes release more micro-particle. Again, silicone is more bio-compatible has a unique defoaming property. A logical balance is hence reached when selecting the tubing for cardiopulmonary bypass, and thus a PVC tube with a silicone inner lining is preferred.

In a roller pump, the column fluid/blood shifts forward as soon as the leading roller head compresses the blood containing tube against the rigid racing track. The minimum amount of blood that can be moved forward in one rotation of the rollers is the column of blood trapped in between the leading and the trailing compressive roller heads. This amounts to:

Diameter of the tube (according to the size of the patient) × Length of tube (between compressive heads)

The pump flow can be increased or decreased by manipulating the rotational speed of the rollers and the amount circulating is maintained according to the physiological needs of the patient. This is continuously monitored and intermittent blood gas analysis and other quantitative tests are done to maintain the milieu intérieur within the physiological range. The control panel has a knob for adjustment of rotational speed, switch for forward and backward movement of the roller, and a small analog panel showing the approximate amount of blood delivered though the oxygenator into the circulation, the direction of flow, and a continuously moving bar showing the amount of flow that very instant. Safety and error messages are displayed as well.

Tubing occlusion is adjusted by a knob attached on top of the roller heads and is considered just adequate when the rate of fall in the water column, open to atmospheric pressure, approximates 1 mm/second. Visual evaluation is normally done even though the industry recommends a more elaborate technique for optimal and reproducible flow. Pump manufacturers recommend setting roller pump occlusion such that the level of a 100 cm column of crystalloid drops by 2.5 cm/min. Prior to this, the roller heads should be in either a 6.00 o'clock or 9.15 o'clock position and the arterial line pressurized to 250 mm of Hg. In practice, the occlusion check is done just prior to joining the arterial and venous ends of the tubing using a connector in a bubble free manner.

OTHER FORWARD FLOW PUMPS

There is only a reference to Dodrill at the Wayne University medical center, Detroit, using the piston-driven pump in cardiopulmonary bypass operations. The pump was constructed by engineers at General Motors and was not considered anymore. The 'finger pumps' that created forward flow came next. The forward movement of the blood column was a result of successive piano keys like compression of the tubing containing the fluid. These pumps were marketed for a time and were effective in the pediatric age-group; the maximum flow possible was 2 liters and thereabouts. The best use of these pumps was noted during Lillehei's 'controlled cross-circulation' times where the pump helped in maintaining a unidirectional and continually flowing circulation.

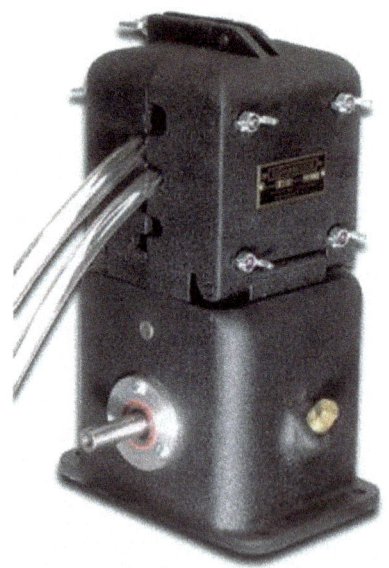

Fig - 21 The Sigma-motor pump

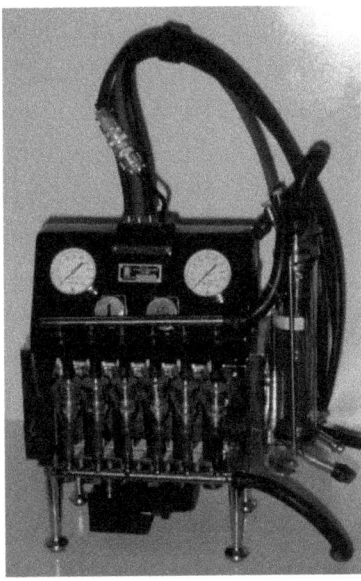

Fg - 22 Dodrill-GMR 'Michigan Heart'

Roller pumps soon became popular and perfusionists and physicians soon realized that this pump was capable of delivering fluid volumes in accordance with a with their choice and the same pump was able to handle both overweight adult and pediatric patients.

CENTRIFUGAL PUMPS

Air/oxygen bubbles and haemolysis were still bothersome and hung a curtain of uncertainty over the safe practice of extracorporeal circulation. Incorporation of defoamers and ultrasonic gas micro-bubble detectors have minimized chances of occurrence of any untoward events. In fact, presence of a micro-bubble in any region of the circuit leads to an immediate stop to the pump. Some degree of haemolysis happens and remains the main problem. The engineers define a centrifugal pump as a mechanical device designed to move a fluid by transferring the rotational energy from one or more driven rotors, called impellers. Fluid enters the rapidly rotating impeller along its axis and is cast out by centrifugal force along its circumference through the vane tip of the impellers. In medical practice and for the construction of a sophisticated heart lung machine, the impeller vanes are made to lie free and pivoted centrally within a hermetically sealed hard transparent shell. Rotational movement occurs by magnetic coupling. Compared with roller pumps, centrifugal pumps offer the advantages of minimising the air pumping potential, less ability to create large positive and negative pressures, less blood trauma, and virtually no spallation. Introduction of magnetic levitation principle for inducing the rotational movement of the impeller vanes magnetic levitation has made the modern cardiopulmonary devices almost noiseless, viz ., the Centrimag and the Levitronix.

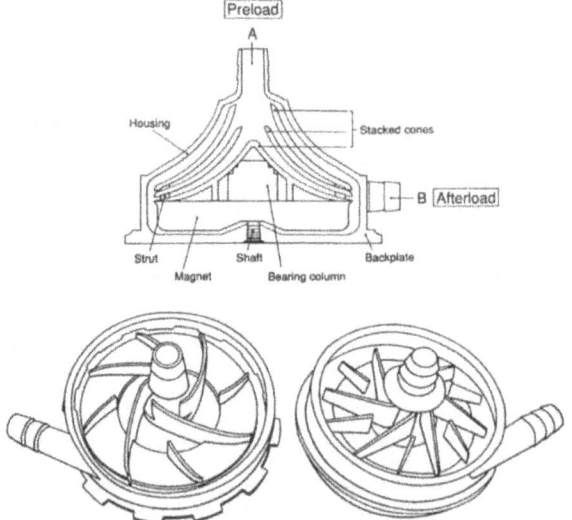

Fig - 23 Centrifugal pump – cross-section & operating scheme

Conventional centrifugal pumps, such as the Biomedicus (Medtronic, Eden Prairie, MN), the Jostra Rotaflow (Maquet Cardiopulmonary, Rastatt, Germany), Revolution (Sorin, Italy), and the Levitronix (Levitronix, Waltham, MA), in addition to the functioning as a heart-lung machine, provide excellent short-term support in extracorporeal membrane oxygenation (ECMO), or as a short-term ventricular assist device (VAD). Direct cannulation is required and a centrifugal pump with a membrane oxygenator is best suited for use > 5-6 hours.

A negative pressure is created at the blood inlet port that leads to an apparent passive drainage of blood sufficient for a centrifugal pump once the rotation of the blades starts. An important issue concerning centrifugal pumps is the dependence of performance on afterload of the patient's circulation.

During cardiopulmonary bypass, be it for a short-term cardiac surgery or extracorporeal support for a longer period, constant blood flow is maintained. The Hagen–Poiseuille equation is relevant here:--

Blood flow rate = Pressure / Resistance

Thus, the pump generates blood flow and pressure against a degree of resistance. Biocompatible material for tubings and other disposable materials are used as for other pumps. Modern pumps have low priming volumes which can be easily controlled and cause less haemolysis. Both are routinely used nowadays and deliver blood over a wide range of flow rates against a variable resistance (resistance across an oxygenator + preload and afterload of the body).

Blood flow in roller pumps depends upon the pump tubing internal diameter, rotation rate of the rollers, and diameter of the pump head.

In centrifugal pumps the centrifugal force generated by the rotating impeller is converted into energy and pressure is generated. Thus:

Centrifugal force = mass × radius × angular velocity

and, in a clinical setting –

Centrifugal force = Mass of blood × radius of pump head × RPM

Centrifugal pumps are totally non-occlusive and a minor variation in pressure in the path may affect the performance. This results in constant fluctuations in blood flow. Therefore, a flow-meter must be incorporated in the arterial line to quantify pump flow. Further, when the pump is not running, blood will flow backwards leading to exsanguination of the patient or aspiration of air. Therefore, when the centrifugal pump is not running, the arterial line must be clamped.

The development of the magnetic levitation technology has made the centrifugal pumps almost noiseless and they are mainly incorporated in the extracorporeal life support systems and transcatheter ventricular assist devices.

CHAPTER – 9
THE PRIME

During the initial period of cardiac surgery, the heart-lung machine with the oxygenator was empirically primed with freshly collected blood (banked blood preserved and anticoagulated earlier with acid citrate-phosphate-dextrose solution that was later upgraded to an even effective citrate-phosphate-dextrose and adenosine solution) to which sodium bicarbonate (as buffer) calcium gluconate (to counter hypocalcemia) and dexamethasone (to reduce the inflammation and as a membrane stabilizing agent) were added. Though reduced flow in low temperatures according to the established *Azygos flow principle* was well known, the belief of that time was:

- Hematocrit had to be maintained,
- De-airing should be meticulous,
- Flow-rate of the bypass machine should be nearly equal to the cardiac output of the patient.
- Dilution, hypothermia and flow sufficient to maintain vital organ perfusion

Ideas and practices have changed since and a perfusionist must always be aware that cardiac operations requiring cardiopulmonary bypass involve a major invasion of the circulatory system of the patient. There are some basic facts that are to be kept in mind before a priming solution for cardiopulmonary bypass is constituted, e.g,--

- The hematocrit should not be below 21% at initiation and 27% during weaning for uneventful recovery,
- Ionic balance of the prime should be approximately equal to that of the normal physiologic range of plasma oncotic pressure,
- Constituent solutions may need to be varied according to the disease or condition the patients might be having,
- Strict asepsis has to be maintained while priming the cardiopulmonary bypass circuit,

The prime is a mixture of a volume of crystalloids and blood to which mannitol and other agents are added. The final volume depends on the size of the patient (body surface area, or BSA), volume of the reservoir + oxygenator + heater/cooler portion, and the length of the circuit integrated with the main pump of the heart-lung machine. Maintenance of Ionic balance and oncotic pressure of the priming volume are major considerations. In adults the usual flow rate is 2.2-2.4 liters/min when ½" tubing is used for venous drainage and ⅜" tubing is utilized in the arterial side and rest.

Low prime volume with miniaturization of bypass circuitry has become popular recently. Positioning of the heart-lung machine close to the patient, placing the main pump as near as possible to the oxygenator, and an assisted drainage (either kinetic or vacuum assisted) for venous return are, individually or together, as the situation demands, found effective in reducing of the foreign surface area to which the blood of the patient is exposed.

Retrograde autologous priming (RAP)/ venous antegrade prime (VAP) is the process of initiation of cardiopulmonary bypass (CPB) to reduce hemodilution. Perfusionists resort to this strategy in selected conditions like severe anemia, heart failure, St. Jehovah's witness, etc. This procedure is the recent choice in acute normovolemic hemodilution and reduces both peri-operative cognitive impairment and the need for blood transfusion thus increasing the hematocrit following cardiac surgery. Near-infrared spectroscopy (NIRS) monitoring or any other method of cerebral oximetry and procedural ultrafiltration aids in acute normovolemic hemodilution and is quite effective in reducing exposure of the blood of the patient to the exterior. However, a universally accepted safe solution is eluding us still and the method of perfusion is individualized, may vary, and quick situational changes may be required. With adoption of a normovolemic low-prime technique, it is safe to withdraw 10-20% of the circulating volume of the patient and replace this with either autologous pre-drawn blood, banked component of blood, or colloids (plasma, albumin or the synthetic ones) and isotonic crystalloids.

The prime volume in cardiopulmonary bypass is a total of the volume needed to fill up the arteriovenous loop of the main circuit plus a reserve volume, or the prime boot, that may be suddenly required in crisis.

The 'diluent' is the isotonic fluid to which various agents like sodium bicarbonate, calcium gluconate dextrose, mannitol, and steroids are used. The amount varies according to the center but the goal is always directed at maintaining biocompatibility, isotonicity, and iso-osmolarity. The volume of diluent is variable. It depends mainly on the type of prime and the type of blood used. In adults, a clear prime is preferred for patients >8-10 kg body weight as long as the hematocrit of the patient is acceptable. Perfusion technologists are more concerned about small babies and blood is used in some form – whole blood and washed banked packed red blood cells. 20% albumin (where available) or plasma is preferred, but 5% dextrose can be used if the body weight is low and the hemoglobin of the patient is relatively high.

The total prime volume is, therefore, an addition of blood and the diluent solution in children. If the body weight is between 6-8 kg, one unit of blood is used.

Again, the diluent in children where approximately 9 gm post-bypass hemoglobin content in the is a target, is as follows:

(Pt. Hb -90)/Pt. Hb x Estimated blood volume of pt.

+ ¼ unit of blood to this makes up the total prime.

It should be remembered that banked blood, in whatever form, contains citrate-phosphate-dextrose as the anticoagulant. Heparinization will be necessary for anticoagulation and a small amount of 5% dextrose, as extra energy substrate, is added in centers where facilities for drawing fresh blood in non-CPD-containing containers are available.

Initiation of bypass may appear routine, but it is crucial. De-aeration should be meticulous and the volume and composition of the prime gives away partially the strategy of hemodilution that is planned. In adults, the team as a whole is afraid of cerebrovascular accidents (CVA) while in babies, the main concern is hypotension.

Key periods during initiation of cardiopulmonary bypass may be summarized as follows:--

Table-V

Initiation of cardiopulmonary bypass (CPB)	Priming, either gravity drainage or vacuum assisted	onset of CPB should be gradual
Heart separated from rest of circulation		
	Control of O$_2$ delivery, CO$_2$ removal relinquished by the anesthetist, and pump flow assumed by perfusionist	Ventilation by anesthetist discontinued
	Mean arterial pressure (MAP) of CPB flow to be adjusted and maintained at a minimum of 50-60 mm of Hg	
		Aortic cross clamp
		Cardioplegia
		Repair/replacement/transplant
		Weaning from CPB & anesthetic ventilation restarted
		Daeration
		Release of cross-clamp & decannulation
		Hemostasis & restoration

The patient operated under cardiopulmonary bypass takes time for respiratory recovery and restoration of autoregulation satisfactory enough for sustenance. Patient transport and maintenance under a ventilator with inotropes and other medicines in the immediate postoperative period are necessary till respiratory and circulatory support can be weaned.

CHAPTER - 10
ADEQUACY OF PERFUSION

The body mass index (BMI) and the body surface area (BSA) have to be calculated or estimated from an appropriate scale by entering the height and weight of the patient. The blood volume of a patient can be roughly measured by these means, and the size of the oxygenator that will be capable of adequate perfusion, is chosen. The vital organs where tissue perfusion is critical are the brain and the kidneys. Neurological parasympathetic autoregulation leading to vasoconstriction would be a problem, but in the anesthetized patient this is not usually a factor. Diabetic patients commonly need an increased perfusion flow.

Adequacy of tissue perfusion by the cardiopulmonary apparatus depends upon many factors. Hematocrit is important though hemodilution to a certain extent is finding favor for better tissue perfusion. Oxygen delivery is dependent on hematocrit - both delivery of oxygen (DO_2) and oxygen combustion (VO_2) are increased when the hematocrit is within a physiologic range. Normal hematocrit values in the unanesthetized and non-cannulated subject are:

- Adult males: 41% to 50%
- Adult females: 36% to 44%
- Infants: 32% to 42%
- Newborns: 45% to 61%

The optimal hematocrit in the prime is taken to be 27%. Lower values, meaning both low DO_2 and VO_2, can be corrected up to a certain value by increasing the pump flow. A low hematocrit is always unwarranted and aside from the morbidity, the patient may not even recover. Prior to the setup of the heart-lung machine, the individuals expected hematocrit in the prime is always calculated as follows:

CALCULATIONS OF PRIME VOLUME FOR THE DESIRED HEMATOCRIT

The steps followed are:

1. Patient's expected blood volume is determined:
   EBV = Patient's Body wt. in kg x Factor^3 (ml/kg)
2. The desired diluted blood volume for cardiopulmonary bypass is calculated: Dilution = Pre-perfusion hematocrit % / Desired hematocrit % during Cardiopulmonary bypass x EBV.
3. The PrimeVolume for the whole circuit:
   Prime volume = Hemodiluted volume - EBV

[The factor varies in accordance with the size of the patient --- Calculation of volume of crystalloid solution (cardiopulmonary bypass prime volume) necessary for hemodilution to a desired hematocrit, estimated blood volume(EBV), and(cardiopulmonary bypass (CPB). Factor (EBV/kg) is assumed to be 80 mL/kg for <10 kg body weight; 75 mL/kg for 10 to 20 kg of body weight; 70 mL/kg for >20 kg of body weight. The example addresses the polycythemic adult, but this condition is more prevalent in cyanotic pediatric patients with smaller required CPB circuit prime volumes].

Adequacy of perfusion can nowadays be assessed by serial lactate, $PaCO_2$, $PvCO_2$, the gradient between arterial and venous CO_2 pressures, and hematocrit levels. Lactate levels when elevated indicate anaerobic metabolism at the tissue level and the lactate-pyruvate ratio is also altered significantly. As a result, there is increased arteriovenous shunting peripherally compounding the perfusion. Though persistent high lactate level is a sensitive marker, it cannot localize the region of hypoperfusion.

Serial measurement of arterial and venous CO_2 saturation by blood sampling and the gradient between the two gives the best idea of tissue perfusion. The normal person beforecardiopulmonary bypass has a PaO_2 of 95 to 100%, and on top of this we are injecting O_2 mixed with air with a blender. Hence, the expected PaO_2 during perfusion is maintained at around anything over 100% and below 120%. This may require a minor tweak of the flow of O_2 at times.

CHAPTER – 11
CARDIOPULMONARY BYPASS — PROCEDURAL DETAILS

SCHEME OF PRE-BYPASS LAYOUT OF THE HEART-LUNG MACHINE

Preparation of the patient and the pre-operative tests, blood and others, are similar to any surgery. Rather, in most cases gut handling is ruled out and intestinal preparations are not required. Though occasional intrusion by an intestinal loop can happen, the operative field will be flooded and obscured by blood if a way to minimize this is not employed. The heart-lung machine provides this opportunity and connecting the patient's circulation to the device with biocompatible cannulas, connectors, and tubings helps the operator to bypass the cardiopulmonary circulation of the patient while perfusing the vital organs. This gives the surgeon valuable procedural time. The actual positioning of the specially designed pump, the venous reservoir, the oxygenator, the filter, the ultrasonic bubble detectors, and connecting the biocompatible tubes between them requires both imagination and logical scientific thinking. In addition, there was the knowledge of the physiological functioning of the human circulation. The idea of isolating the circulation is according to the following scheme:

PLAN OF CARDIOPULMONARY BYPASS

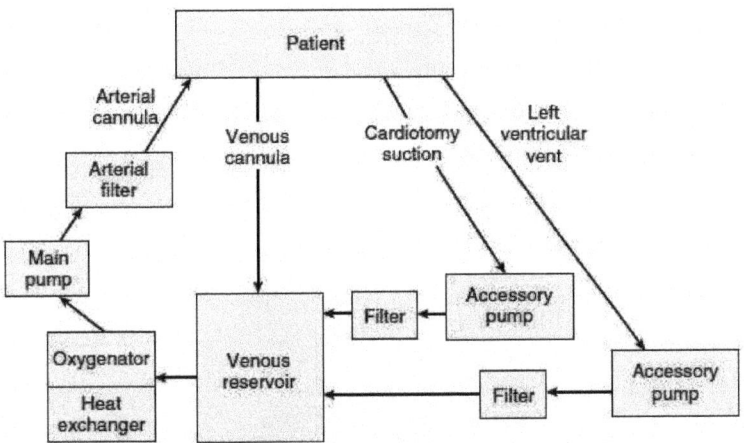

The position of the pump varies according to the type of oxygenator used. The recent hollow fiber and membrane oxygenators are resistant to blood flow from the venous reservoir. Added to this will be the resistance of the patient and the arterial filter. The body's circulatory resistance is physiologically known as the Systemic Vascular Resistance (SVR) and to this is added the pressure drop across the oxygenator and the arterial filter. Together the resistance is insurmountable and so requires a pump to be placed in between the venous reservoir and the oxygenator-heat exchanger complex so blood and plasma can flow freely and the circulatory flow is unidirectional and unimpeded. In practice while setting up cardiopulmonary bypass an accessory pump and a filter are not used to keep matters simple. Vents are important to prevent ventricular distension and the following reasons are also important:-

1. Delay myocardial rewarming,
2. Help to keep the operative field dry,

3. The aortic root vent minimizes the chance of air embolism to the brain.

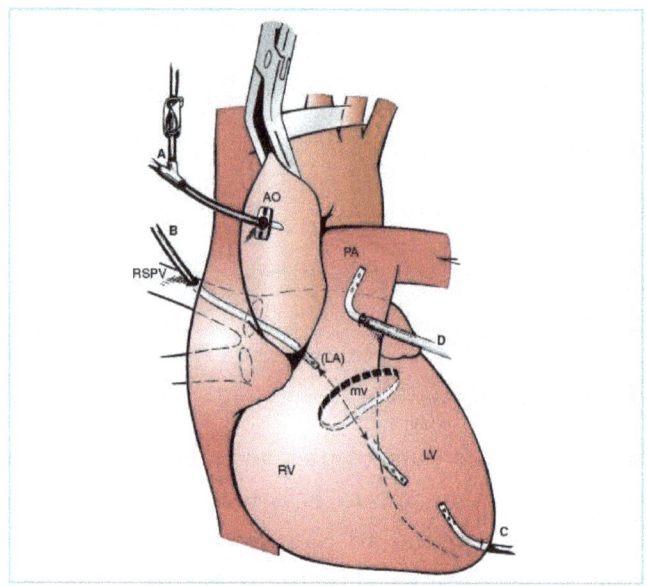

Fig - 24 Common venting sites

The preferred venting sites are:

- Right superior pulmonary vein →mitral valve →left ventricle,
- Main pulmonary artery,
- Aortic root using the cardioplegia cannula.

The majority depend on vent introduction before application of the cross-clamp. This comes with a risk of air introduction that can be avoided if precautionary measures are taken. Pulmonary artery venting is indirect and safe if a shunt can be ruled out. Apart from a cardioplegia cannula (and its variants), the LV vent cannula is a long malleable PVC tube with multiple side holes and an end hole and with a malleable metallic probe for guiding it through the mitral valve into the LV.

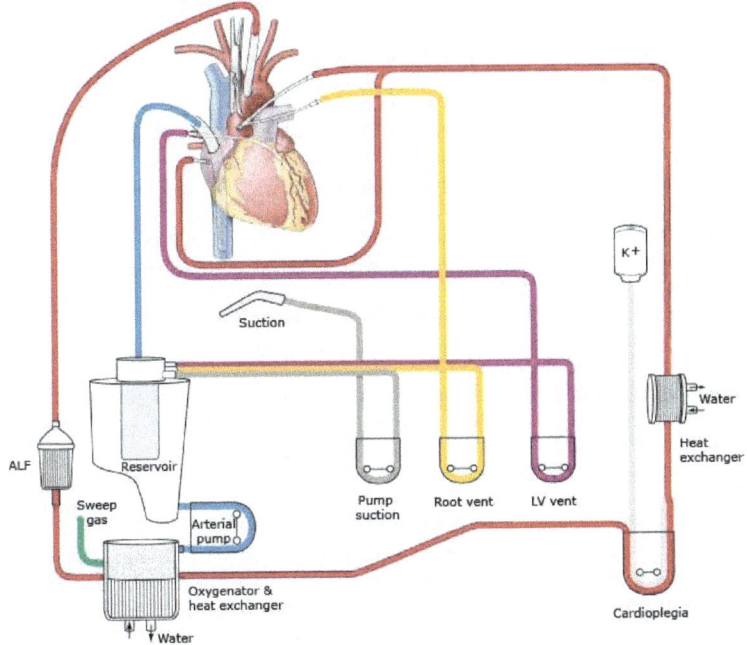

Fig - 25 Schematic Diagram of Cardiopulmonary Bypass

In addition there may be a purge line between the oxygenator and the venous reservoir with a manifold in the line mainly for sampling.

The above is a schematic diagram of the cardiopulmonary bypass system when hollow-fiber or membrane oxygenators are used.

Filters are used both inside a venous reservoir and in the arterial phase just after the oxygenator for the blood to circulate in the patient's systemic circuit. These minimize the chances of gaseous and particulate embolism. Venous and arterial filters are of 120 µm and 40 µm mesh size, respectively. The filter on the venous side is integrated with the reservoir, while a separate and dedicated arterial filter has to be attached to the tubing after the oxygenator.

CONDUCT OF CARDIOPULMONARY BYPASS

Lillehei was a maverick and wild; Kirklin, on the other hand, was disciplined. A separate station for setting up the heart-lung machine was the practice since then following Kirklin's practice. Effort was made to keep the tubing length as short as possible, minimizing the chance of generalized inflammation due to exposure of blood to a large external surface. The first important step was positioning the heart-lung machine with respect to the patient. This primarily gives the approximate length of the tubes needed for arterial and venous sides. The larger the drainage tubing diameter, the better is the venous drainage and studies are there to show 1 cm venous drainage is better but a ½" tube diameter is the largest diameter available and usually used in 70 kg adults for a gravity venous drainage from the body to the reservoir. The compressive roller heads and their rigid racing track are constructed with ½" and ⅜" tubing, commonly used in the roller pumps. In practice, ½" internal diameter (ID) tube is used for venous drainage, ⅜" ID tubings for arterial flow, and ¼" ID tubes used in pediatric patients and small babies. The ¼" tubings are also used for cardiotomy suction, vent, and cardioplegia. Reversal of the cardioplegia line will start a slow suction pressure aiding de-aeration further before release of cross clamp.

The ½" tubing from the body, connected via a Y-connector to single or double stage venous cannulas draining venous blood from the right atrium/SVC & IVC, is attached to the designated port in the reservoir. Next a length of 3/8" continuous tubing is taken for attachment to the venous reservoir at one end, placed in sockets and positioned snugly alongside the rigid backing track with the leading and trailing compressing roller heads. The other end of the tubing is attached to the inlet port of the oxygenator. The heart-lung pump unit also has a holder for the modern-day combination of venous reservoir and oxygenator with heating-cooling systems. This is a set-up used in the main pump.

Length of ¼" tubings are used for:

1. Cardiotomy suction,
2. Vents, and
3. Cardioplegia.

The accessory pumps in the console are utilized for these.

Any operative procedure on the heart on cardiopulmonary bypass will incite some inflammatory response and the operative field requires constant clearance of residual bleeding for proper visualization. The suction port of the cardiotomy suckers are designed and constructed to minimize hemolysis and retrieve blood which would otherwise have been lost and help to maintain an appropriate hemoglobin concentration and reduce the need for homologous blood transfusions. Cardiotomy suction employs a gentle negative suction by one of the natural, accessory pumps in the heart-lung machine console and the surgical team is seldom aware of the gentleness required for handling this. Studies have conclusively shown that the blood sucked by cardiotomy suction is more inflammatory and loaded with Tumor necrosis factor (TNF), TNF-α, complements, and microaggregates. The slightest contact with pericardial fluid heightens this effect and in centers where a cell-saver is available, heparin coating of the flowing surface together with washing and a re-infusion of the shed blood salvaged by suction minimizes –

1. Lowering of hematocrit.
2. Pathophysiological effects of a deranged coagulation cascade.
3. Eliminates the deranged platelets of shed blood, and most importantly
4. Minimizes hemolysis.

Vent suction should be slow and steady. Too strong suction may lead to a collapse of the cardiac walls of the chamber where the vent cannula is introduced into. In dire states, one may resort to trans-septal venting, and this can be an effective ploy to avert a bad situation.

Cardioplegia is essential during cardiac surgery as a paralyzed and supple heart is needed for correction and placement of sutures. Cardioplegia infusion is commonly prepared and infused with an accessory pump by a perfusionist as a volume of 300-500 ml at the rate of 200 ml/min is required for an arrested heart in the adult. The route and type is chosen by the surgeon, but the perfusionist should have an idea of the nature of surgery that is going to be performed and the timed repetitions of the cardioplegic solution that will have to be made. Many types of cardioplegic solutions are in the market, e.g., clear crystalloid fluids, St. Thomas' solution, cold and warm blood in crystalloid fluid (1:4), and the single dose cardioplegic solutions (similar to Bretschneider or the Kerr solutions). The Kole chamber (disposable/reusable) was solely used for drawing and reconstituting early versions of crystalloid and blood cardioplegia that had to be repeated every 15-20 minutes. Of late the single dose solutions are preferred – industry manufactured Custodiol HTK (matching intracellular ionic concentration) and on-table prepared Del Nido solution (matching extracellular ionic environment). The latter was prepared specifically for myocardial protection in small babies and infants. The DelNido solution works well with adults as well. The single dose cardioplegic solutions are preferred because the duration of surgical arrest is prolonged and interruptions are few if any at all. Moreover, the contractile recovery appears better with less evidence of the ill effects of anaerobic metabolism or reperfusion.

CHAPTER - 12
RECENT IDEAS & ADDITIONAL TECHNOLOGICAL APPLICATIONS

While conducting a cardiopulmonary bypass, one frequently comes across the terms 'mini-bypass' and 'microplegia'. Mini bypass is basically concerned with minimizing exposure of circulatory blood to the external surface. This entails shortening of tubes of venous drainage and arterial lines, vacuum assisted venous drainage, integration of a venous bubble filter within the reservoir, and incorporation of the oxygenator with heater-cooler along with the reservoir.

This entails a reorientation of apparatus and kinetic venous autologous priming as well along with the use of a two stage heart-lung machine also helps. Research shows that the institution of these measures causes a definite reduction of the magnitude of the systemic inflammatory response incited after an operation under cardiopulmonary bypass. The modern day perfusionists now routinely conduct mini bypasses for better outcome during cardiac surgery under cardiopulmonary bypass.

Microplegia was proposed to improve myocardial protection, minimization of tissue anaerobic metabolism with production of lactates and superoxides, and a reduction in cardioplegic volume with better maintenance of the post-bypass hematocrit. Microplegia essentially has to be blood cardioplegia with 66:1 proportion of blood and other clear fluid ratio while in conventional cardioplegia the proportion is only 4:1. Extensive studies were performed between the various types of cardioplegia and there was little difference among the various types with respect to induction of arrest, recovery of spontaneous rhythm, and incidence of arrhythmias in the post-bypass period. Moreover such a solution required frequent and timely injection. This concept never became popular.

PULSATILITY

Physicians & surgeons are accustomed to see a pulsatile pulse tracing synchronized with the electrocardiogram and the heart rate. So it is obvious that there will be fascination for pulsatile waves generated by the heart-lung machine and a belief that the pulsatile wave in the circulatory system will be good for tissue perfusion. The heart-lung machines used daily produce mainly a non-pulsatile flow that appears as a saw-tooth continuous line. However, studies so far have not been statistically significant and there are no pulsatile waves in the capillaries. The pumps, both the roller and centrifugal, can be engineered to propulse fluid in a pulsatile fashion. As the benefit is minimal, if any at all, the prohibitive cost escalation precludes the use of such modified pumps.

ULTRAFILTRATION

This modality is a relatively newer procedural addition to cardiopulmonary bypass and was introduced in 1976. There are two primary reasons:-

1) volume management, and
2) mediator-removal.

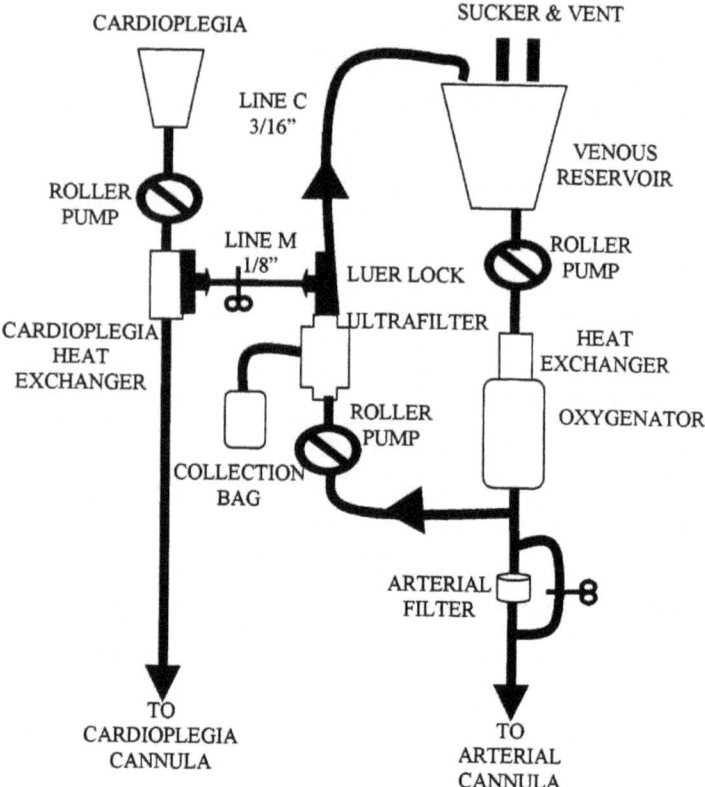

Fig - 25 The accompanying diagram is a scheme for conventional continuous ultrafiltration technique (CUF) during cardiopulmonary bypass.

Conventional ultrafiltration (CUF) and modified ultrafiltration (MUF) are common in cardiopulmonary bypass today. CUF is carried out during cardiopulmonary bypass to maintain moderate hemodilution and minimal venous reservoir blood, and MUF can be performed after discontinuation of bypass and is used routinely of late, as MUF gives the patient an extra advantage by removing the inflammatory markers.

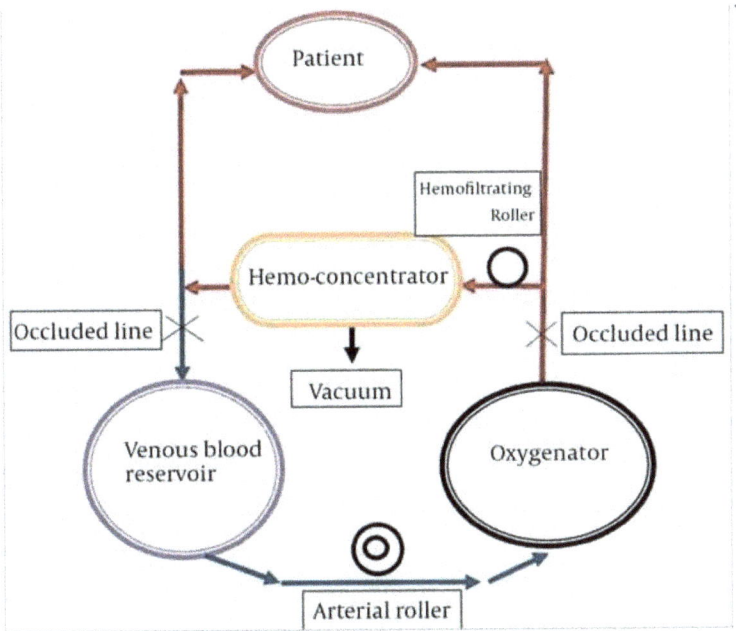

Fig - 26 Schematic diagram of the MUF.

Post-operative patient recovery is better with modified ultrafiltration (MUF) than in those not receiving any ultrafiltration at all. Dedicated hemofilters or hemo-concentrators, as they are called, can be purchased, but a simple dialyzing membrane does the same job cheaply and is sufficient. The ultrafilter membrane has a pore size of 0.01 nm and selectively filters out the harmful substances including bacterial and viral pathogens. Whatever be the adjunct, the goal is zero-balance ultrafiltration (ZBUF) with the aim of not adding any extra fluid during cardiopulmonary bypass.

CHAPTER - 13
MONITORING DURING CARDIOPULMONARY BYPASS

Nowadays we find a patient wired to several monitors and the number has been increasing day by day as physicians try to gather as much information as possible, especially those having some form of external manifestation. This helps to keep the patients physiological mechanisms within an acceptable range. It has to be understood that in the early days of cardiac surgery under cardiopulmonary bypass, there were no methods to know the central venous pressure, no facility for doing frequent blood gas analyses, and the team could not even think of continuous blood pressure recordings. Digital palpation of the superficial temporal artery by the anesthetist, who had to insinuate his hand under the drapes, was the only sign available. Minimally invasive modified Seldinger techniques of radial artery and internal jugular/subclavian cannulations have armed the treating team to be aware of :--

1. Pulse & continuous blood pressure from which the mean arterial pressure can be calculated,
2. Sampling ports for frequent & serial blood gas & electrolyte measurements,
3. Anesthetic drug injection directly into the heart for induction and maintenance,
4. Direct right atrial continuous infusion of inotropes, vasodilators, and other medicines for immediate action in required situations,

5. Continuous measurement of the central venous pressure and thus being aware of roughly the volume status and the right sided pressures of the heart,
6. The central venous pressure tracing shown in the monitor is an important indicator of right sided cardiac function, especially atrial contractility and movement of the atrioventricular valves with systole and diastole.

Additionally, along with the ECG, the venous pulse wave reveals arrhythmias and are indicative of atrioventricular dissociation.

In fact, the pulsatile depiction of a continuous arterial pulse in a crude oscilloscope and viewing a continuous real time ECG were the first monitors available. Gradually new parameters like central venous pressure, pulse oximetry (SpO_2), respiratory rate and pattern, surface and core temperatures, and end-tidal respiratory CO_2 ($ETCO_2$) were added and could be viewed in a single window of the screen of the monitor.

Impending or sudden occurrence of untoward events could now be diagnosed and treated quicker with a better outcome and a fall in the mortality rate.

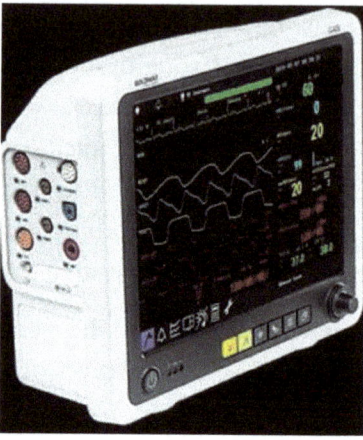

Figure-27. Multichannel Monitor.

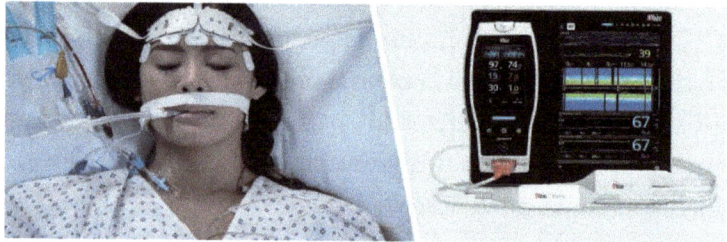

Figure-28 NIRS cerebral oximetry.

Prevention of ischemia of the neural tissue of the brain and spinal cord is a major issue in major aortic surgery like aneurysms and dissections. Prolonged operative time, extensive dissection, and interruption of spinal vessels are all significant. Measures adopted include intravenous pentothal, profound hypothermia, and cerebral perfusion when deep hypothermic arrest is preferred. Controlled cerebrospinal (CSF) drainage by a lumbar puncture to keep the CSF pressure on the lower side is also done. While the bispectral index (BIS) helps anesthetists to monitor the depth of anesthesia and the efficacy of the stroke volume as long as it is beating, cerebral oximetry by near-infrared spectroscopy (NIRS) is the choice during cardiopulmonary bypass. NIRS reflects hemoglobin saturation in venous, and capillary blood in brain tissue as it indicates oxygenation by absorption of the reflected infrared light. It is noninvasive, and the monitor can be used throughout a prolonged procedure and also in the postoperative period in heart and vascular surgeries. Early measures like a flow increase (↑MAP) and normalizing blood $PaCO_2$ levels by adjusting the gas sweep by the perfusionist may salvage the situation when the cerebral saturation is falling.

Monitoring continuous cardiac output (CO) has now been added and the present methods used in the available monitors include either the continuous thermodilution method (CCO) or a continuous estimation of the area under the curve and contour of the arterial pulse wave (pulse contour cardiac output - PCCO). The minimally-invasive FloTrac system helps advanced hemodynamic monitoring by automatically calculating key flow parameters every 20 seconds. A continuous clarity is provided and a decision to manage the hemodynamic instability accordingly.

The anesthetists, nowadays, insist upon routine end-tidal CO_2 ($ETCO_2$) monitoring. This not only gives the assurance of the correct position of the endotracheal tube, but the characteristic box-shaped curve with the permissible score roughly indicates arterial CO_2 and the adequacy of perfusion. The appearance of unwarranted spikes in the curve is consistent with the patient's own inspiratory effort and lightening of anesthesia.

Of late, some industry leaders have been integrating continuous in-line monitoring with spectrophotometric optical fluorescence and reflectance-based systems. These monitors continuously monitor up to 11 critical blood gas parameters with lab-quality accuracy. The sensor is placed around the blood-filled tubing of the CPB circuit and allows measurement of pH, PCO_2, O_2, K^+, PaO_2, hematocrit, hemoglobin, and temperature. The initial cost of such heart-lung machines are high.

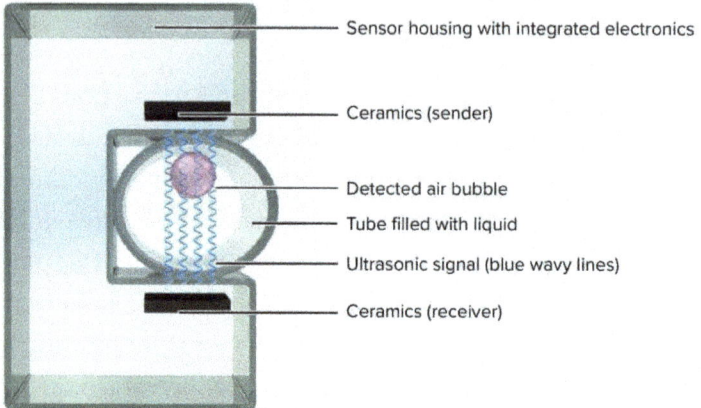

Fig - 29 A bubble Sensor

The heart-lung machines recently are being provided with a clip-on ultrasonic bubble sensor which can additionally quantify the flow. This non-contact technology maintains sterility and uses two piezoelectric crystals, one a projector of the ultrasonic beam and the other a receiver or sensor. The change in the impedance sets off an alarm and stops the flow.

Other sophisticated appliances like an oxygenation sensor for the blood inside the tube to be transfused or a macro-bubble sensor just after the venous reservoir may augment the safety, but these are not used widely and make little difference when not.

- The operation theater in cardiac surgery is a crowded place. In addition to the surgical team and the nurses (at least one scrub nurse and a floor nurse), members of anesthesia and perfusion are essential. The anesthesia machine with its built-in ventilator and the monitors take up much of the space. The heart-lung machine is bulky. The console has a main pump (roller or centrifugal), at least three other roller pumps, the reservoir-oxygenator-heater/cooler with the holder, and the cardioplegia delivery system are clubbed together and have to be closely adjacent to the patient. Wires and tubing from and to the body of the patient, the heart-lung machine, the monitor, and the anesthesia machine with its respirator can be found at multiple places in the operating room. These are seen:
- on the floor (mainly water for heaters and coolers, pasted with lengths of adhesive tapes),
- at waist height and thereabout (mainly tubing between the patient and the heart-lung machine and the oxygenator, and leads to the monitors),
- from the gas and suction ports on the wall.

The anesthesia machine and the ventilator tubing are at the head end of the patient. In addition, there is a defibrillator and the bulky hemotherm apparatus. Proper placement and organization are essential so that personnel can operate an appliance if the situation warrants. The patient is made to lie on a ripple mattress (with circulating air or water) and the legs with the calf muscles encased in intermittent and sequential compression stockings. These measures minimize the incidence of pressure sores and deep vein thrombosis. In rare situations an intra-aortic balloon pump (IABP) or an assist device (ventricular assist device [VAD] or extracorporeal membrane oxygenation [ECMO]) may be needed to maintain organ perfusion and space has to be made for the appliance with its accessories. During the early days the gadgets were not so numerous, but with a large oxygen cylinder, air compressor, buckets of ice, and 1 to 1.5 HP Tullu type pumps, the scene was even more chaotic.

This is how a recent cardiac operating room with the heart-lung machine and a seated perfusionist looks like.

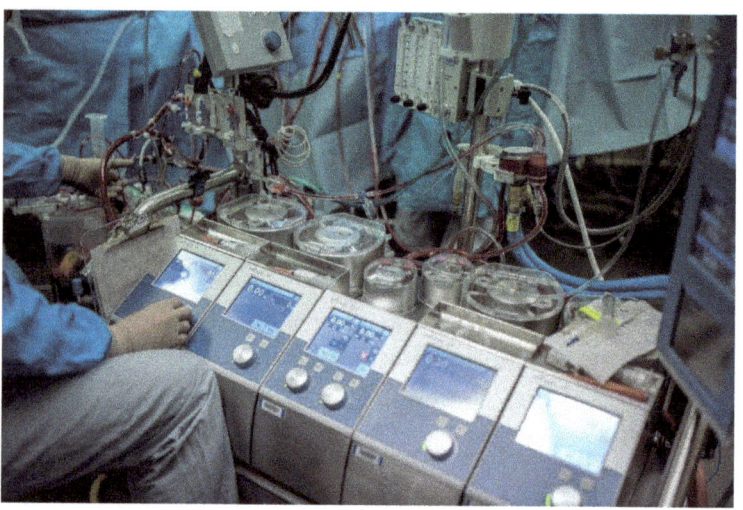

Figure-30 Perfusionist and the heart lung machine.

CHAPTER – 14
GASSES USED IN CARDIOPULMONARY BYPASS

The primary role of the oxygenator is to act as the surrogate of lungs for a period as near to physiology as possible. We, humans, breathe in environmental air containing roughly 21% of O_2. Nitrogen constitutes 78% and the rest is a mixture with Argon making up the majority. These environmental gasses behave the same way inside the body as they should outside and obey all the laws of physics pertaining to gasses. Another important thing is that O_2 and CO_2 transport in the lungs do not follow a linear relationship. The process of oxygenation differs from CO_2 removal and has a very complex interrelation – increasing ventilation thus increases both oxygenation and carbon dioxide removal in areas of the lung removal where the ventilation/perfusion (V/Q) is maintained. On the other hand areas of low V/Q there is a preferential increase in O_2 uptake compared to CO_2. The blender adjusts the gas mixture, oxygen and compressed air. Increasing the flow rate of the heart-lung machine will lead to an increased flow through the oxygenator, that is devoid of the auto correction capability unique to the living. The fraction of inspired oxygen (FiO_2) is always maintained so that the partial pressure of arterial oxygen remains at 100-150 at the normal flow rates of 2.2-2.4/liter per m^2 of BSA in the adult and proportionately less in patients with lower body weight. Actually, the PaO2 level is always kept hyperoxic and the $PaCO_2$, which is considered more important, should never be above 45.

After cardiopulmonary bypass the ventilatory capacity of the patient and the consequential gas transport is altered. The patient empirically is provided ventilatory support till the gas transport system corrects, the patient can generate a spontaneous breath, and the muscle power is satisfactory enough to sustain the respiratory power of the patient.

pH MAINTENANCE

The most common way of looking at blood gas analysis reports during an ongoing cardiopulmonary bypass is sampling blood in a heparinized syringe directly from a manifold that is attached with a thin tubing at designated ports in the main bypass circuitry. The blood gas analyzers lately are miniaturized and provide comparable reports in real time in the operating room. For the majority the α-stat method where immediate analysis results of the circulating blood concerning its acid-base, ionic, HCO^{3-}, anion gap, etc, are shown and corrections made accordingly.

The pH-stat method needs a correction factor for the temperature for the real-time actual values to be shown. Though studies to date have failed to show a difference in clinical outcome, still there is a belief in some that cerebral blood flow during hypothermic states or deep hypothermic arrest the pH stat strategy gives a more reliable scene of the cerebral blood flow.

CHAPTER – 15
CARDIOPULMONARY BYPASS IN THE PEDIATRIC PATIENT

Cardiopulmonary bypass in small children is challenging and there are some special problems unique to babies. Small children should never be considered as miniature adults and scaling down a problem is never a solution. Both water content and skin surface area are proportionally higher in babies in comparison with adult patients and the principal areas needing focus when perfusion is concerned are:

1. The organ systems are evolving and still are not mature,
2. The organs are small requiring delicate handling,
3. The circulatory system with the vessel size and diameters is considerably small,
4. The circulating volume is also on the lower side,
5. O_2 consumption is high,
6. The pulmonary vascular tree is reactive and a small change can lead to major adverse issues,
7. Intra- and extra-cardiac shunts may take time to close especially in premature infants. In fact such shunts may be protective in some complex congenital conditions,
8. The child's heart tolerates ischemia better,
9. Temperature control is poor.
10. An early change of the oxygenator may be in order due to a poor tolerance to embolic insult.

Though theoretically speaking 7 gm/dl Hb of the child is considered a cutout value for hemodilution of prime, most centers are comfortable with 8-9 gm/dl of Hb. BSA nomogram and the Dubois formula are used for calculations.

The estimated blood volume, as calculated, will be approximately–

> 10 Kg — 85 ml/kg,

10-20 Kg - 80 ml/kg, and

21-45 Kg - 75 ml/kg.

The calculated cardiopulmonary bypass flow rates vary, and flow rates in total bypass at 37^0 are recommended as follows –

- 3kg and less – 150-200 ml/kg/min, 3-7 kg - 120-190 ml/kg/min,
- 7-10 kg - 100-170 ml/kg/min,
- 10-30 kg - 80-100 ml/kg/min, and
- 30-50 kg - 75-100 ml/kg/min.

It is interesting to note that the flow rates decrease with an increase in body weight and approach the normal rate after 45 kg.

The minimum predicted flow rate for a small heart in most centers is <1500 ml/min on full bypass requiring a total prime volume, including the arterial and venous lines with the boot, of approximately 350 ml. Practically, the size and type of the arterial line and the cannula depend on visual estimation and the comfort of the surgeon. The operating room should have 1/4" (8Fr), 3/16" (10Fr), and 1/8" (12Fr) tubings and appropriate cannula (according to the surgeon's choice) for arterial lines. At the same time one must remember, the smaller the internal diameter of the tubing greater will be the circulatory resistance and the optimum hemodynamic energy will not be delivered during perfusion. The venous line in small babies is usually 3/8th of an inch up to 3 kg of body weight. The arterial line tubing will be 1/4" for body weight of 1500 gms to 2 kg. Most centers still use gravity for venous drainage. 3/8" tubings are used in all places, e.g. arterial, venous, and boot lines when the weight of the baby varies between 2-3 kgs. At and above 3 kg body weight, 1/2" drainage lines are used while the arterial line remains at 3/8". In addition, the perfusion team of various centers where infant complex congenital repair is done, have individualized protocols with subtle differences. Periodic handouts are posted on the Net for facilitation of members. Recently further small sized oxygenators for infants (prime volume as low as 31 ml) and tubing internal diameters of 5/32" have been developed. These together with the incorporation of two levels of two centrifugal pumps (one main pump and the other for kinetic or vacuum-assisted venous drainage) and close on-table placement of the oxygenator reduce both the priming volume and tubing length considerably.

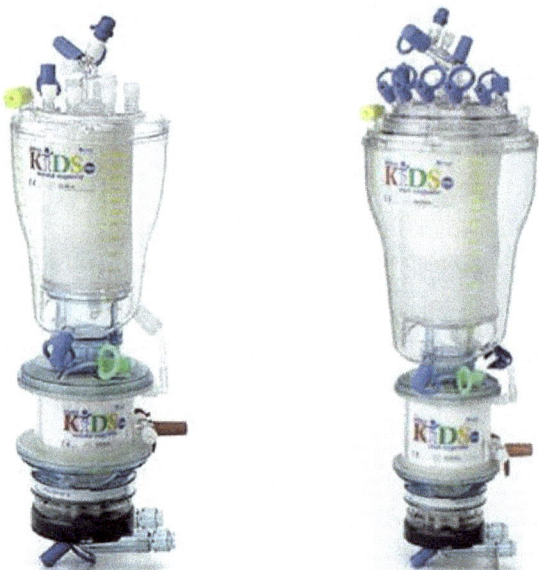

Fig - 31 Oxygenators for babies

Perfusionists are wary of hypotensive and extreme hemodilution (vary from 50-200%) at the initiation of bypass and stick to a fixed protocol for reproducible results. A blood-primed cardiopulmonary bypass circuit is frequently necessary and pump-flow is adjusted to maintain a mean arterial pressure of 20-70 mm of Hg to prevent these events.

The minimum temperature to which the pediatric patient can be lowered during bypass should not be below 18^0C. Most of the relatively short-lasting operations are done at 28^0C. Both α-stat and pH-stat methods are employed for maintenance of acid-base balance.

Children have a high metabolic turnover and the oxygen combustion measured is about 6-8 ml/kg. Like adults, the O_2 saturation in children hovers around 95-100%. The difference in children is that the saturation is FiO_2 dependent and nitric oxide may have to be blended for the reactive vascular bed. Periodic blood gas analysis gives both the partial pressures of O_2 and CO_2 as the best parameters for monitoring the gas levels. Normally gas blending is done in such a way that –

- Oxygen levels are always hyperoxic obviating any chance of hypoxic episodes,
- Flow of O_2 acts as a 'sweep' for CO_2 during the countercurrent gas flow through the hollow fiber oxygenator,
- PaO_2 should not be >200 so that oxygen induced lung injury does not happen,
- The range of $PaCO_2$ varies from 20-60, in difference to the narrow range of 35-45 in adults.

All centers use a nomogram for body surface area (BSA) determination.

For further simplification, pediatric cardiac surgical teams divide patients into two groups ≤ 10 kgs and >10 kg body weight. Babies < 10 kg will have a flow rate of about body weight times 150 ml/min/kg. In pediatric patients above 10 kg body weight, the flow rate is calculated in a different manner and this approximates to 2400 ml/M^2/min. Simplification is made with the necessity of blood as well – 100 ml is used when the age of the infant is 6 months or less, 90 ml between 6 to 18 months, and 80 ml after 18 months of age.

Safe bypass in small children is fraught with uncertainties and the entire surgery not only aims at anatomical correction but also a full cognitive and functional recovery. Initiation of bypass should be slow and a steady mean arterial pressure (MAP) of >50-60 mm Hg is steadily maintained. Temperature changes have to be cautiously monitored as the regulatory center in the brain is not mature. A minimum gradient of 8^0C must always be there between the core temperature and that of blood, especially during rewarming. Intermittent blood gas sampling is done to find out the pH and ionic status and the activated clotting time (ACT) for heparin anticoagulation. The number of such samplings is to be kept at a minimum though some such samplings must be done at timed intervals. Nevertheless, blood sampling in a heparin-rinsed syringe should be done whenever there is a doubt.

CHAPTER -16
THERMOREGULATION

TEMPERATURE MANAGEMENT IN CARDIO-PULMONARY BYPASS & OPERATIONS UNDER DEEP HYPOTHERMIC CARDIAC ARREST

Temperature management became an integral part of operations under cardiopulmonary bypass after Bigelow's seminal experiments on hibernating animals in cold temperature. There was even a period in the 20th century, '70s to '90s, when space scientists became interested in the possibility of induced human hibernation in space laboratories. Realization of the fact that there is a fall in the metabolic rate proportional to the body temperature after a phase in general anesthesia, made cardiac surgeons use temperature reduction as an adjunct organ protective tool in cardiopulmonary bypass and cardioplegic arrest.

Thermoregulation in the living body is complex, and this figure is a simplistic representation of the events that happen and how hypothalamic regulatory centers manage this --

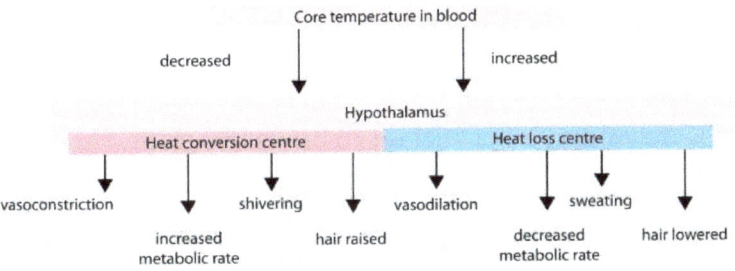

Fig – 32: Temperature regulation in the body

Hypothermia in the anesthetic patient is, however, different. Three distinct phases have been identified – a) phase-I when redistribution of the temperature due to vasodilatation, b) phase-II linear reduction of heat loss and core temperature falls below the temperature of other parts of the body, and c) phase-III the equilibrium phase where a thermoregulated generalized vasoconstriction is there and the heat loss can be matched by the metabolic production.

By a complex mechanism there is proportional decrease of the cardiac tissue oxygen consumption and the brain is also protected. The various levels of hypothermia are :--

- Mild Hypothermia, 95-89.6°F/35-32°C
- Moderate Hypothermia, 89.6-82.4° F/32-28°C.
- Severe Hypothermia, 82.4-75.2°F/28-24°C
- Suspended animation or Apparent Death, 75.2-59°F/24-15°C.
- Death from irreversible hypothermia.

In cardiac surgery under cardiopulmonary bypass the benefits are:

1. Extension of the operative time.
2. Myocardial protection
3. Cerebral and other vital organ protection, and
4. Lessening the chance of infection.
5. Reduction in bleeding in the operative field.

During cardiac surgery, the above mentioned rigid 5 stages of hypothermia are not observed and for practical reasons the simplified division below is followed:

1. Mild - 37° to 35° C.
2. Moderate - 35° to 28° C, and
3. Severe -28° C and less.
4. Profound - <24°C or according to some <20°C

DEEP HYPOTHERMIC CIRCULATORY ARREST (DHCA)

The majority of the cases are done in the temperature range of 35-28°C. Deep hypothermic circulatory arrest (DHCA) is needed in major vascular surgery and dissection and control of bleeding in certain difficult situations. These are desperate conditions with dire consequences and surgical palliative repair is the only hope and DHCA is done knowing fully that cognitive recovery may not be entirely as before. Satisfactory neural recovery occurs when the arrest time does not exceed 40 minutes.

Relatively bloodless fields and long operative time in complex defects warrant deep hypothermic circulatory arrest (DHCA). In complex neonatal or infants' periods of DHCA is induced as and when needed both for facilitating the repair and better cognitive recovery. DHCA is practiced in the narrow range of 20° to 16° Celsius (C). The recent trend has been an antegrade or retrograde cerebral flow in addition to a period of DHCA for better cognitive recovery.

In 1963 in South Africa, Barnard and Schrire were first documented to use DHCA to repair an aortic aneurysm.

Cooling the patient to 10°C. and stopping the circulation for a period R. B. Griepp, in 1975, is generally credited with demonstrating DHCA as a safe and practical approach for aortic arch surgery. DHCA is never a panacea, rather the modality is a leap into the unknown. During the period of circulatory arrest tissue perfusion does not occur and consequently the question of oxygen consumption does not arise. The anesthetists inject cerebroprotective doses of thiopental (59%), propofol (29%), and others (48%). Of the others, corticosteroids, though controversial, are commonest. Both these drugs cause "burst suppression" and deepen the plane of anesthesia. Though thiopental is known for a dose dependent myocardial depression, both have smooth and timed reversal effects. Other agents used depend upon the idea and belief of the team doing the surgery and may consist of any or a combination of the following:

- Calcium channel blockers,
- Protease inhibitors (aprotinin, nafamostat),
- Free radical scavengers (mannitol, desferrioxamine),
- Amino acid receptor antagonists (magnesium),
- Glutamate release inhibitors (lidocaine, fosphenytoin), and thromboxane A_2 receptor blockers, etc .

Steroids may induce raised blood sugar levels and a control with insulin is required. An event-free EEG or a quite somatosensory potential was often advised in the past, but has not proved worthwhile with time.

Operative time may be prolonged by combining DHCA with selective antegrade carotid arterial or retrograde venous cerebral perfusion. The complexity of surgery is increased by both the methods. As superior vena cava (SVC) is cannulated most of the time and as the cerebral veins do not have any valves, a retrograde venous perfusion with 200-500 ml/kg/min is adequate in perfusing the cerebral tissue. This route is preferred in emergency situations and combat of suspected intraoperative air embolism. Selective arterial perfusion is usually an elective procedure and specialized cannula, that are usually balloon tipped, are used for the carotids on either side. A flow of 10-20 ml/kg/min is required. In both the methods the MAP should be maintained at 50-60 mm of Hg. The temperature can hover between $22\text{-}25^0$ Celsius and further lowering to $18\text{-}20^0$ C is not required.

DHCA is primarily considered for safety of the brain. At normothermia, brain injury has been observed after 4 minutes of circulatory arrest and cerebral metabolism is said to decrease by 6–7% for every 1°C drop in temperature from 37°C and thus there is a reduction in oxygen consumption by the neural cells in the brain. Circulatory arrest is undertaken at 18–20°C and a range of safe periods for DHCA have been reported at this temperature. 30 minutes of DHCA have been found to be safe without significant neurological dysfunction. There is an increase in the incidence of brain injury after 40 minutes and beyond 60 minutes, the majority of patients will have irreversible brain injury. A small number of patients tolerate longer periods but the numbers are not predictable. Neonates and infants compared with adults have been found to tolerate longer periods but due to the unpredictability, 40 minutes is universally accepted as the safe period.

There is little to monitor during a relatively quiet phase of DHCA. A transcranial Doppler has been found to be least affected by the temperature change and various electromagnetic waves and can be used. A constant watch is necessary so that the arterial wave never shows a MAP below 50-60 mm Hg. The core and surface temperatures require separate monitoring. Finally, time monitoring should be considered most important.

Blood-gas analysis should be done periodically and pH-stat correction and interpretation tends to give best acid-base and electrolyte results matching the physiology of the cells at that particular period.

CHAPTER – 17
ANTICOAGULATION IN CARDIOPULMONARY BYPASS & ITS REVERSAL

ANTICOAGULATION

Anticoagulation in patients having cardiac surgery under cardiopulmonary bypass is a contentious issue. Till date there has been no replacement for unfractionated heparin (discovered in 1916). The usual effective dose of heparin is recommended as follows: Initial dose: At least 150 units/kg; frequently, 300 units/kg is used for procedures estimated to last less than 60 minutes or 400 units/kg for those estimated to last longer than 60 minutes. Unfractionated heparin has erratic behavior and is unpredictable. The estimated half-life ranges from 60-90 minutes.

In practice, the first dose of heparin is injected directly, at the patient's right atrium by the surgeon or into the central port of the central venous line, just before aortic cannulation (MAP approx. 90-100 mm Hg). A customary wait for 3 minutes is usual or a wait for a blood sample drawn after heparin injection and the customary wait period shows a activated clotting time (ACT) value of 480 seconds (clinically accepted range >300-500 secs.). Heparin takes at least 3 cardiac cycles to uniformly mix with blood in the circulatory system, and hence the 3 minute wait.

Dosage in cardiac surgery is on the higher side and not a one-time affair. A full therapeutic dose of Heparin sodium capable of continuous maintenance of an activated clotting time (ACT) of 480 seconds is now considered adequate. Intravenous heparin is available in many forms, e.g. 1000 units per mL, 5000 units per mL, and 10,000 units per mL; these can be used for IM or s.q. Each mL of commercial heparin (5,000 Units per mL) preparation contains: 5, heparin Units 5 mg sodium chloride; 1.5 mg methyl-paraben; 0.15 mg propyl-paraben; Water for Injection q.s., Made isotonic with sodium chloride. Pediatric patients often require a higher dose of heparin and a dose in the following manner is accepted worldwide:

Initial Dose: 75 to 100 units/kg (intravenous bolus over 10 minutes)

Maintenance Dose Infants: 25 to 30 units/kg/hour; Infants < 2 months have the highest requirements (average 28 units/kg/hour)

Children > 1 year of age: 18 to 20 units/kg/hour; Older children may require less heparin, similar to weight-adjusted adult dosage.

Standard sequence for anticoagulation management for adults undergoing CPB:

1. Arterial blood sample for baseline ACT
2. Unfractionated heparin inoculated via central venous catheter
3. Blood sample for ACT after 3–5 min
4. Ensure ACT above 3–4 times of baseline ACT (>480 seconds)

5. 5000-10,000 IU unfractionated heparin to the CPB prime solution.
6. Monitor ACT at least every 30 min during cardiopulmonary bypass
7. Maintain ACT 400–480 seconds during hypothermia while on CPB (24–30°C).
8. Reverse heparin with protamine after separation from CPB. (Dose ratio 1 mg protamine per 10 IU of heparin, based on pre-CPB heparin dose).

The prime is also heparinized to match the patient's circulation and an initial amount of 5000 IU (earlier) to10,000 IU (of late) is injected into the prime when adult patients are considered. One third of the first dose is injected after 90 minutes and, thereafter, repeated every 30 minutes of extra bypass time. This strategy has been found to maintain a steady ACT level of 480 seconds.

It has to be mentioned here that though ACT is used to monitor the level of anticoagulation in cardiopulmonary bypass, measurement of anti-Xa levels may be more accurate. However, studies still support ACT evaluation with an auto-analyzer.

Gravlee et al suggested a dose of 300-400 IU/kg for both the patient and the prime. This maintained the ACT above 480 seconds. This is optimum and in addition to lessening the burden of microclot formation within the bypass circuit such a dose also lowers the chance of hemorrhagic episodes in the patient's organs.

Research has shown adequate anticoagulation at 300-400 seconds of ACT, but stray clots cannot be ruled out and hence the additional dose and the recommended 480 seconds of ACT.

Earlier the perfusion protocols depended on fixed weight-based heparinization during cardiopulmonary bypass. This consisted of 3-4 mg/kg body weight injected directly into the patient's body and 1 ml (i.e.5000 IU) to the prime. ACT was done manually with a pinch of diatomaceous earth or kaolin clay and a cardboard covered light bulb with the top open. The test tube containing the blood was agitated with fingers in the heat emanating from the light bulb. A stop-watch gave the time required for coagulation to occur. Later studies and availability of ACT analyzers in the operating room made frequent measurement of the clotting time and maintenance of anticoagulation for cardiopulmonary bypass easier.

Though the use of heparin is universal in all cardiovascular cases, problems may rarely happen in rare cases, e.g.:

- Heparin-induced thrombocytopenia – In rare situations, the platelet count may drastically fall below 1 lakh/mm^3,
- Once in a while the patient may show an unusual resistance to the administered heparin. Heparin resistance can be multifactorial. Excessive platelet count, deranged antithrombin activity, and heparin-induced thrombocytopenia (HIT-I and HIT-II) are usually dreaded. Of these HIT-II is the most dangerous as it leads to formation of microemboli and can lead to microembolisms and gas exchange disorders with increased resistance to blood flow through oxygenators,
- Recent findings suggest a peculiar resistance to heparin and rise in the levels of other proinflammatory factors with COVID-19 infection.

If at any time the ACT appears to be below the recommended value of 480 seconds, measures are taken. Most situations resolve with the injection of an additional dose of heparin (1 ml or 5000 IU) into the perfusate and infusion of fresh frozen plasma. In the US, FDA-approved antithrombin concentrate is available and its infusion may specifically resolve the situation more quickly.

In certain situations, heparin anticoagulation cannot be used. The reasons are usually allergy and extreme intolerance to additional heparin, heparin-induced thrombocytopenia and thrombosis (HITT), excessive hemodilution, etc. Alternative strategies include the use of recently manufactured direct thrombin inhibitors like r-Hirudin, Bivalirudin, Argatroban, Tirofiban and the relatively new Nafamostat mesilate. However, all of these have short half-lives and require frequent administration. The antithrombin inhibitor Dabigatran and the factor Xa inhibitors (apixaban, edoxaban, and rivaroxaban) are now guideline recommended to reduce the risk of thrombotic events in patients with atrial fibrillation (AF). These later-developed newer anticoagulants are oral agents and preferred post-PTCA stenting by cardiologists.

Heparin is still the first choice in CPB and in very rare situations an alternative has to be considered. The same applies for reversal with Protamine.

REVERSAL OF ANTICOAGULATION

Once the operation is completed, reversal of anticoagulation becomes important for achieving satisfactory hemostasis before sternal apposition and wound closure. As said before, heparin is usually used for anticoagulation in surgeries under cardiopulmonary bypass and protamine is used for reversal of heparin-induced anticoagulation.

In the early periods of cardiovascular surgery, in the 1950s and early '60s hexadimethrine bromide (Polybrene) was used for anticoagulation reversal. Reports of renal failure in dogs made the surgeons queasy and protamine sulfate, extracted either from salmon sperm or produced by genetic recombination, replaced this agent. The onset of action of protamine sulfate is approximately 5 minutes. The agent is available in injectable water solution in 250 mg vials and 10 mg is in 1 ml. The product monograph mentions: "Protamine Sulfate Injection, is a sterile, isotonic solution of protamine sulfate. It acts as a heparin antagonist and a weak anticoagulant. Each mL contains: Protamine sulfate 10 mg; sodium chloride 9 mg; Water for Injection. Sulfuric acid and/or dibasic sodium phosphate (heptahydrate) may have been added for pH adjustment. No preservatives are added and once brought from storage, should be immediately used.

When administered alone, protamine has an anticoagulant effect. However, when it is given in the presence of heparin (which is strongly acidic), a stable salt is formed and the anticoagulant activity of both drugs is lost. Protamine sulfate has a rapid onset of action and 1 mg of protamine sulfate neutralizes 100 IU of heparin. The quantity of protamine sulfate to be injected can therefore, calculated from the total amount of heparin injected. Neutralization of heparin occurs within five minutes after intravenous administration of an appropriate dose of protamine sulfate.

Protamine has certain drawbacks and specific measures have to be taken quickly to overcome these unwanted effects.

Diabetics on NPH (Neutral Protamine Hagedorn) insulin, patients allergic to fish, pregnant women, nursing women, children, those with previous protamine exposure and men who have had vasectomies are considered to have a higher risk. The drug should be injected slowly as rapid injection can lead to cardiovascular collapse due to a sudden vasodilatation. Other severe reactions consist of anaphylactic reaction and severe pulmonary vasoconstriction. The definitive measures may be summarized as below:

A. Primary measures:

- Stop protamine administration
- Maintain airway with 100% O_2
- Stop all inhalational anesthetics
- Start intravascular volume expansion with crystalloid, colloid or blood
- 500 mg to 1.0 g calcium chloride
- 0.1 to 1.0 mg epinephrine IV bolus
- May use pacemaker, ephedrine or atropine when bradycardia complicates the situation
- Phenylephrine 50-100 mcg IV bolus if there is hypotension only
- Reinstitute cardiopulmonary bypass in refractory conditions

B. Secondary measures:

- Antihistamines may be given prior to protamine administration:
- Catecholamine infusions:
- Aminophylline

- Corticosteroids in the form of hydrocortisone during the rewarming phase.

In high risk conditions and patients back on bypass:

1. After loading with steroids, discontinue CPB. Modified Ultrafiltration should be very effective for this patient to remove cytokines and activated complements prior to attempting heparin reversal for the second time..
2. Heparin reversal may be attempted or allowed to be broken down over time, with the ACT returning to normal naturally.
3. Protamine may be given by the surgeon into the left atrium, allowing dilution and dissemination systemically prior to the AT III-Heparin-Protamine complexes entering the pulmonary vascular system.
4. Concomitant Calcium Chloride administration may be useful.

There are a few alternatives to heparin-induced anticoagulation in cardiac surgery under cardiopulmonary bypass. We know that heparin naturally exists in circulation and it is the fine balance between the heparin antithrombin interaction which maintains a clot-free circulatory environment. It is the additional heparin injected, for anticoagulation during cardiopulmonary bypass, that requires neutralization.

In vascular and other surgeries, injected heparin is not neutralized and if bleeding is not a problem the patient recovers without any untoward events. If a cell-saver is available or if following weaning from bypass, the heart appears edematous, reversal is not contemplated and the shed blood, once washed and centrifuged, is re-infused along with other colloid and crystalloids with the goal of maintaining viable mean arterial pressure with acceptable hemoglobin levels for organ perfusion.

Knowing the half-life and metabolism of heparin, it is expected that the action of excess heparin will wear off by 2-4 hours. Known protamine sulfate alternatives are recombinant platelet factor P4 (Intravenous rPF4) and the recombinant inactive antithrombin (rAT). Though these are used in the US, their availability in the operating room is a problem and the cost is prohibitive. As a result, surgical teams continue to use protamine sulfate only for the present and reverse the heparin-induced anticoagulation with a nervous expectation of nothing happening.

CHAPTER - 18
ARTERIAL BLOOD GAS AND THE PERFUSIONIST

Heart surgery under cardiopulmonary bypass is a mammoth exercise where both circulatory function of the native heart and the gas exchange ability of the lungs are completely taken over by a device. To maintain the 'milieu interior' within physiological ranges the whole team should be conversant with normal values of partial pressure of gases, electrolytes, lactates, hematocrit, pH, etc. for comparison. A blood gas analyzer provides these values within a very short time and arterial samples are drawn at intervals so that necessary corrections are possible. Before the start of cardiopulmonary bypass or a connection to the heart-lung machine and the oxygenator, arterial blood sampling is done directly from the arterial port of the patient. Once bypass starts with visual stabilization of MAP and hematocrit, sampling of the oxygenated blood is done by the perfusion team from a manifold attached to a purge line in front of the heart-lung machine.

At the beginning of cardiac surgery under cardiopulmonary bypass, measures were taken relying on certain prefixed ideas and assumptions. Subsequent research, expansion of knowledge, and the development of sophisticated analyzers helped better understand what is happening within the body of the patient. First the bulky reagent based blood gas analyzers were introduced, which additionally measured the bicarbonate levels. Na^+ and K^+ levels were provided after the operation and at the end of the day by the laboratory personnel by using the sample in a flame photometer.

The multi-channel monitors and the bulky reagent based arterial blood-gas and electrolyte analyzers helped the team to add agents or make subtle changes just after a detailed report was available. Miniaturization and cartridge-based blood gas analyzers led to a further improvement and the same parameters were not only portable and cheap but could be carried into the O.T. or ICU. Statistically significant variation is not seen when compared with the bulky reagent-based analyzers.

The usual parameters on arterial blood-gas and electrolyte analysis depend on the cartridge used and the basic parameters are : —

1. pH, 7.35 to 7.45.
2. Pa_{O_2} 95-100 mm of Hg with a Fi_{O_2} of 0.21.
3. Pa_{CO_2} 35-45 mm of Hg with a Fi_{O_2} of 0.21.
4. Hb% 14 to 18 g/dl for males; 12 to 16 g/dl for females.
5. HCO^{3-} 22-26 mEq, varies according to pH and Pa_{CO_2}
6. BE -2 to +2 mEq/l.
7. Na^+ 135-145 mEq/l.
8. K^+ 3.4-4.6 mEq/l.
9. Cl^- 96 to 106 mEq/l.

The perfusion team should be aware of the normal values and try to maintain within the normal range and concentrate on the dynamic task of running a viable circulation and gas exchange by altering the flow rate of the heart lung machine and fraction of gas flow through the blender. The figure that follows indicates in simplified terms the acid-base status of the body and corrections are made accordingly. During operation under cardiopulmonary bypass, both gas exchange and circulation are controlled. Corrections are minimally needed. Infusion of whole blood or packed red cells takes care of low hematocrit and an acidic situation is managed by half correction of the base deficit by the addition of a measured amount of 8.4% sodium bicarbonate.

Table - VI

DISORDER	pH	[H⁺]	PRIMARY DISTURBANCE	SECONDARY RESPONSE
METABOLIC ACIDOSIS	⇓	⇑	⇑HCO_3^-	⇑pCO_2
METABOLIC ALKALOSIS	⇑	⇓	⇑HCO_3^-	⇑pCO_2
RESPIRATORY ACIDOSIS	⇓	⇑	⇑pCO_2	⇑HCO_3^-
RESPIRATORY ALKALOSIS	⇑	⇓	⇑pCO_2	⇑HCO_3^-

This is a simple table that helps in forming an idea of the basic abnormalities that characterize the acid-base disorders. Stress is given to HCO_3^- and pCO2 levels and efforts are made with sodium bicarbonate added to the circulating volume for correction.

Full correction dose of $NaHCO_3$ (mmol) = 0.3 x base deficit (mmol/L) x wt (kg)

Initially a half correction is done with the expectation that the intrinsic circulatory buffer system will take over and make the necessary changes. Further additions depend upon the physician's discretion. Alterations in the sodium level do not require any correction. Normal urine production ensures a normal electrolyte and acid-base balance. Concern about the potassium level is justified in beating heart conditions. Hypokalemia suggested by a blunted and short T-wave and corroborated by an ABG report, can be corrected with the addition of injection potassium chloride (20%). The team is more concerned about hyperkalemia during the weaning period and until rhythmic cardiac contractions in the post-recovery period supervenes. It should be remembered, however, that this hyperkalemia is intracellular and can cause a sudden cardiac arrest from which recovery is difficult. Immediate measures consist of the correction of acidosis and administration of calcium injection.

At the outset, the perfusionist should check whether the arterial-alveolar O_2 gradient is acceptable. This provides a clue to the hypoxemia and abnormalities in gas exchange as the arterial-alveolar $(a - A)$ gradient (calculated by subtracting PaO_2 from PAO_2) is an index of the efficiency of oxygen uptake in the lungs and under normal physiological conditions is < 2.0 kPa.

Another term the perfusionist should be aware of is the anion gap. This in simple terms is the difference-or gap-between the negatively charged and positively charged ionic electrolytes in your blood. The perfusionist most often does not have to do anything about this.

CHAPTER – 19
TROUBLESHOOTING

Sudden and unexpected complications can happen anytime during an intracardiac repair under cardiopulmonary bypass and problems may individually affect surgeons, anesthetists or be perfusion related. The fact is that all the members of the team should be aware of these issues, but the onus of finding a quick solution is always on the perfusionist. The dreaded complications and the possible solutions are: –

1. Sudden drop in venous drainage.
2. Leak in connector or tubing.
3. Oxygenator change during a procedure.
4. Sudden intraoperative air embolism of the brain.
4. Target vessel for arterial cannulation is too small.

Most of these problems have been observed in practice seen and successfully managed. Human error accounts for the majority of the disturbances and simple corrective measures help to overcome these situations. Major power failure can be catastrophic which is why a hand-crank is included with the roller pumps.

PROBLEMS WITH VENOUS DRAINAGE

When there is a sudden drop in venous return or when the venous return is not satisfactory, the surgeon instinctively tries to lower the venous reservoir level and checks the position of the tip of the inferior vena cava cannula that has been introduced through the right atrium. Gravity venous drainage is the chosen method most of the time and an increase in the siphon gradient is theorized to increase the return.

Due to anatomical variations, hepatic vein drainage may be blocked and a slight or gradual withdrawal of the cannula solves the problem in the majority of the cases. This problem is mainly seen with snug-fitting, two-stage venous cannula. In bicaval cannulation this is a problem after the venous snuggers are in place. Releasing of the IVC snugger followed by withdrawing the cannula as far as practical—keeping all the holes of the cannula with a short length for snugging—resolves the issue in most cases.

Core temperature reduction should be started simultaneously. When the actual procedure is expected to be a short one, a confident surgeon may quickly proceed and complete the procedure, instructing the perfusion team to manage under a low-return low-flow condition while maintaining a lower temperature. However, the low venous return has to be steady. At the same time, it should be understood that adding clear fluids in such a condition increases hemodilution, further compromising the oxygen-carrying capacity of circulating blood may be precarious. If volume needs replenishment, administering blood is the only answer.

It is mandatory that the whole team understands that cardiopulmonary bypass is now carried out with a low priming-volume setup and vacuum assisted venous drainage is used only in pediatric cardiac surgery. Deep hypothermic arrest with retrograde cerebral circulation is only considered in extreme situations.

The perfusion team should also watch for and prevent excessive venous drainage. In this situation the inner venous walls wrap around the cannula in such a way that the draining holes are intermittently occluded. Venous drainage is not satisfactory or steady. The condition is commonly seen with vacuum assisted venous drainage requiring a decrease in the suction force. The condition is also known in cardiopulmonary bypass as "cavitation".

A large venous cannula will lead to a collapse of the inferior vena cava and right atrium around the cannula. This is seen as "chatter" in the venous line with poor venous drainage and congestion of the lower part of the body. The resultant venous hypertension may even lead to renal damage.

There should be no holes in the venous cannula that are exposed to atmospheric air once the right atrium is opened. This inadvertently leads to an air-lock in the venous drainage line and if height manipulation fails to drive the trapped column of air out of the drainage tube, cerebral protective measures such as crushed ice around the patient's head, intravenous pentothal and steroids have to be given along with a complete cessation of the pump for a short period. During this period the affected cannula is pushed further in to ensure no hole is exposed, a clamp is placed on the venous cannula, the venous drainage tubing is clamped just below the air column and it is then filled with an isotonic fluid minimizing air as far as possible. Finally the cannula and the drainage line are reconnected as before. Cardiopulmonary bypass can now be resumed with the release of clamps.

DEFECTS IN TUBINGS & CONNECTORS

Safety in cardiac surgery under cardiopulmonary bypass is like walking on thin ice. Accidents can happen at any time and from unexpected quarters. Theoretically air embolism from the venous side can reach the arterial portion of the tubing, however, this rarely happens due to a number of filters, bubble detectors and traps. Air bubbles in the venous drainage tube are easier to manage and can be removed rapidly without the fear of cognitive complications.

An escaped bubble into the circulation from the arterial system is ominous and if the brain is affected, a loss of cognitive response after the reversal of anesthesia may be noticed. Redundancy of tubing length may make things easier by sectioning the affected portion as required and then rejoining the two ends together with a connector. The primed filled tube needs to be clamped at both the ends, and the reconnection has to be air-free. A connector with a Leuer side port helps with deaeration.

Leaking connectors are dealt with similarly.

A small leak in the tubing, on the drainage side or on the forward flow side can be identified by the continuous trickle of the prime flowing inside. The first reaction is the application of a liberal amount of bone wax to block the leak. If the procedure is of a short duration and the surgeon is confident, no other measures are necessary. A larger hole poses the risk of suction of a large bubble by the 'Venturi' effect. In roller pumps, there is a term called 'spalling' where microaggregates of tubing material may enter the circulation due to the continued wear by the compressive heads within the racetrack. If by chance a part of the wall of the tubing is weak, a fracture may occur in this part. In this case the leakage is bigger and a temporary stoppage of the pump, institution of full cerebral protective measures, anesthetic lung ventilation with an FIO_2 of 1 followed by a change of the tubing within the pump should be done.

CEREBRAL AIR EMBOLISM

There is a saying that "air in the head and the patient is dead". A strong degree of suspicion is required to presume embolization to the brain. Immediate measures have to be taken to decrease the effect and extent of brain damage.

The question that comes to mind whenever a cardiac surgery patient fails to regain consciousness is 'How much air in the bubble form is relevant'? It is well-nigh impossible to eradicate all microbubbles in the bypass circuitry and when a sizable air bubble escapes into the brain, oxygen-containing blood to that region of neural tissue is cut-off by an 'ink-bottle' phenomenon, blocking the minute capillaries. Air in the bubble is absorbed within hours, but by this time, neural tissue dies. Symptoms depend upon the region affected, and even entrainment of a tiny bubble may be fatal. The affliction of unimportant areas may be associated with irritability and the subsequent control may necessitate prolonged ventilation with a quiet patient in a head-down and left-side up position (Durant position). Reduction of the core temperature, in addition, is advised. On the operating table, the patient lies supine with wires of several gadgets attached and so a left-side-up position is not possible quickly. With the availability of hydraulic operating tables, the quick assumption of a steep head down position, i.e, the Trendelenburg position, is possible.

It is advised at this point that time is important and a quick remedy limits the neurological damage.

OXYGENATOR CHANGE OUT

Nowadays, the stakes in cardiac surgery are high, and a failing oxygenator is a potentially fatal complication. A liberal estimate mentions 1 oxygenator related problem for every batch of industrially made oxygenators. Most are discarded before use, and only in a rare case where problems arise during a procedure, is immediate change is warranted to restore oxygenation and to prevent embolizations. The possibility of this occurring should always be considered and the members of the team have to work sequentially with the goal of resuming normal cardiopulmonary bypass as early as possible. There are two techniques of oxygenator change out during a procedure: –

1. The classical, time-consuming method, and
2. The recently proposed "pronto" technique.

The classical method is followed mostly for two reasons – first, the avoidance of the additional cost burden, and second, nobody wants to waste something costly since a defect in the oxygenator is rare and it is even rarer to develop during the critical stage of the procedure. The steps for oxygenator change using the usual method with a roller pump consists in:

1. Maneuvers to decrease the body temperature are to be initiated immediately, The Hemotherm machine helps and also maintains the safe temperature gradient.
2. Crushed ice should be placed surrounding and in contact with the head.

3. A new oxygenator should be attached to the holder replacing the defective one. The gas, water, and matched tubing for venous inflow and post pump outflow should be quickly attached. The arteriovenous loop reformed.
4. The arterial tubing is quickly threaded along the racetrack and the compressive head of the rollers.
5. Priming is rapidly done using larger caliber tubes and needles, if required.
6. Deaeration is performed with an arterial filter in the circuit.
7. Arterial and venous tubings should be reconnected with fresh connectors and the pump should be restarted.

Nowadays a simpler and less time consuming protocol is followed and this consists in –

1. Water lines and disconnected from the oxygenator.
2. Tubings to the defective oxygenator is liberally swabbed with alcohol and then severed between clamps. The defective oxygenator is discarded.
3. A new oxygenator is retrieved from its package.
4. Lengths of appropriate-sized tubing are attached to the oxygenator and clamped.
5. Bypass is discontinued and the arterial and venous lines are clamped towards the patient side.
6. The AV bridge is opened and a new oxygenator is inserted and connected below the bridge with connectors. A crystalloid prime is started immediately.
7. Deaeration is done through the AV bridge.
8. Gas and water lines are re-attached to the new oxygenator.

9. The AV bridge is clamped and the pump is started again.

Needless to say, temperature reduction should go on simultaneously and cerebral protective measures are to be instituted to the fullest.

With the COVID pandemic there has been an exponential rise in the use of ECMO. In such conditions a change of the oxygenator becomes mandatory after a few days. The big units with affluent patients make it a practice to have a clamped spare oxygenator in a bridge so that the pump requires minimal stoppage. This is the 'pronto' technique, and since its introduction, it has been essential for complex pediatric practice and extracorporeal life support systems (ECLS), but seldom used for adult intracardiac repairs.

CENTRIFUGAL PUMP DEFECTS

These pumps, despite their superiority, are not as robust as roller pumps. On rare occasions the centrifugal pump may suddenly fail or develop functional defects. This change may be fecilitated if a bridge with tubing is there beforehand. This technique is valid for intracardiac repair cases and has not been tested with the more sophisticated newer ECMO devices which integrate the pump and the PMP hollow fiber oxygenator.

PROBLEMS WITH VESSEL CANNULATION

It must be remembered that in cardiopulmonary bypass the major vessels require leak-proof cannulation. The possibility of dissection, atherosclerotic embolization, and a sudden gush of bleeding cannot be ruled out. Precautionary measures are taken accordingly and a pre-procedural epiaortic ultrasonographic scan may be done, if the facility is there, for determining the nature of the aortic wall. In the majority of cases, venous cannulation is done through the atria. Venous walls are usually thin and supple and the main concern is proper intracavitary cannula insertion without separation of the walls ensuring adequate venous drainage. A practical solution is applying two opposing stay sutures and then pulling them apart just before making a clean and bold incision within the purse-string suture on the anterior wall of the vein. The tip and the side holes of the venous cannula are introduced and guided into the venous cavity and a column of deoxygenated blood, approximately equaling the central venous pressure, is visualized. The problem is most commonly seen with direct venous cannulation by novices mostly.

An aortic cannula has a narrowed portion which is inserted into the vessel lumen and there is conventionally an end hole. The prime enters the aorta at a considerable pressure and the narrowing of the cannula at this region leads to increased velocity of flow of the prime. If the cannula tip faces a wall of the aorta, there is the distinct probability of thinning of that portion of the aortic wall due to the constant 'sandblasting' by the prime. This weakened and thinned out wall is a possible site for aneurysm formation.

Alternative cannulation sites should always be kept in mind and if the target arterial diameter appears to be small, a biosynthetic graft may be sutured end-to-side. The arterial cannula is introduced into the graft and securely tied. The method has certain advantages, viz.: a) flow is bi-directional negating ischemia of the distal part, and b) 'sandblast' injury is prevented.

CHAPTER - 20
CONCLUSION

Cardiopulmonary bypass was initially developed to facilitate cardiac surgery. With the advancement in therapeutic methods new durable and leak-proof gas exchange membranes and membrane-like oxygenators were developed. The aims were complete postoperative cognitive and functional recovery, safe cardiopulmonary bypass (especially in small babies) and post-repair improvement in quality of life.

Intracardiac repair under cardiopulmonary bypass is a matter of a few hours. The same principle is applied in the extracorporeal life support system (e.g, ECMO and $ECCO_2R$) which may last for extended hours. Patients usually require these late in the course of illness, either for the failing heart or the lungs. These may be used long-term, sometimes for days, weeks or even months, and the time of weaning can never be predicted. Veno-venous ECMO has been used successfully as a bridge to transplant or recovery. The COVID pandemic saw extensive use of ECMO with the goal of salvaging patients and a minor modification of the gas-transferring medium allowed enhanced CO_2 washout. Studies are in progress and ECMO and $ECCO_2R$ are broad subjects beyond the scope of this write-up.

Intracardiac repair and cardiopulmonary bypass are interrelated. The work of the perfusionist in managing the resources at their disposal along with the heart-lung machine and the oxygenator requires some degree of knowledge and expertise. This compilation is an effort to answer the frequently asked questions that the senior perfusionist or a cardiac surgeon faces every time they work.

REFERENCES

1. https://www.rbht.nhs.uk/blog/history-cardiac-surgery.
2. https://pubmed.ncbi.nlm.nih.gov/2205175/.
3. https://www.ncbi.nlm.nih.gov/pmc/articles/PMC8360707/.
4. https://www.physio-pedia.com/Lung_Volumes.
5. https://mrmjournal.biomedcentral.com/articles/10.1186/s40248-017-0084-5.
6. https://pvrinstitute.org/media/4060/pulmcircchap2.pdf.
7. https://resources.wfsahq.org/atotw/respiratory-physiology-part-2/.
8. https://www.sciencedirect.com/science/article/pii/S0735109722004648.
9. https://www.ahajournals.org/doi/10.1161/circ.102.suppl_4.IV-87.
10. https://www.ahajournals.org/doi/10.1161/CIRCULATIONAHA.108.830174.
11. https://www.ncbi.nlm.nih.gov/pmc/articles/PMC6936302/.
12. https://www.ncbi.nlm.nih.gov/pmc/articles/PMC4813537/.
13. https://www.researchgate.net/figure/Hollow-fiber-membrane-oxygenator-Fresh-gas-called-sweep-runs-through-the-center-of-the_fig2_350424739.
14. https://anesthesia.bidmc.harvard.edu/ADEL/Documents/Cardiac/CARDIOPULMONARY%20BYPASS.pdf.
15. https://www.rch.org.au/uploadedfiles/main/content/cardiac_surg/perf2004.pdf.
16. https://www.annalsthoracicsurgery.org/article/S0003-4975(09)01582-3/pdf.
17. https://www.ncbi.nlm.nih.gov/pmc/articles/PMC5613602/.
18. https://www.uptodate.com/contents/management-of-cardiopulmonary-bypass.
19. https://www.thieme-connect.com/products/ejournals/pdf/10.1055/s-0039-1700529.pdf.
20. https://academic.oup.com/ejcts/article/33/3/418/359278.
21. https://www.ncbi.nlm.nih.gov/pmc/articles/PMC4557578/.
22. https://pubmed.ncbi.nlm.nih.gov/33043657/.
23. https://pubmed.ncbi.nlm.nih.gov/23561819/ .

24. Cooley DA. Tex Heart Inst J. 1999. PMID: 10524736 Free
a. PMC article.
25. https://associationofanaesthetists-publications.onlinelibrary.wiley.com/doi/10.1111/j.1365-2044.2006.04781.x.
26. https://academic.oup.com/icvts/article/3/4/535/676624.
27. https://www.annalsthoracicsurgery.org/article/S0003-4975(03)01820-4/pdf.
28. https://pubs.acs.org/doi/pdf/10.1021/ba-1973-0118.ch001.
29. https://www.mdpi.com/2077-0375/10/11/362.
30. https://www.ncbi.nlm.nih.gov/pmc/articles/PMC5683297/.
31. https://www.ncbi.nlm.nih.gov/pmc/articles/PMC10010948/.
32. https://www.jtcvs.org/article/S0022-5223(19)38052-3/pdf.
33. https://pubmed.ncbi.nlm.nih.gov/21719530/.
34. https://thoracickey.com/cardiopulmonary-bypass/.
35. https://daily.jstor.org/the-decapitation-experiments-of-jean-cesar-legallois/.
36. https://www.bjcvs.org/article/2832/en-us/Hemolysis-and-Inflammatory-Response-to-Extracorporeal-Circulation------during-On-Pump-CABG--Comparison-between-Roller-and-Centrifugal-Pump------System.
37. https://www.sciencedirect.com/topics/nursing-and-health-professions/centrifugal-pump.
38. https://www.sciencedirect.com/science/article/abs/pii/S1053077097901099.
39. https://www.ncbi.nlm.nih.gov/pmc/articles/PMC59
40. https://www.ncbi.nlm.nih.gov/pmc/articles/PMC4680762/.
41. https://www.tsda.org/wp-content/uploads/2012/12/CPB_Skills_Print_Version.pdf.
42. https://www.sciencedirect.com/science/article/pii/S1743181617303414?via%3Dihub.
43. https://www.ncbi.nlm.nih.gov/pmc/articles/PMC3963732/.
44. https://academic.oup.com/bjaed/article/10/5/138/274654.

BOOKS CONSULTED

1. Taylor KM editor 1986: Cardiopulmonary bypass, principles and management.
2. Cardiovascular Perfusion: A Comprehensive Guide To Studying for, and Passing, the American Board of 3. 3. Cardiovascular Perfusion Examinations, Nathan Spitz.
4. The manual of clinical perfusion, 2nd edition, Lich & Brown.
5. Perfusion for congenital heart disease, Gregory S. Matte.
6. Cardiopulmonary Bypass and Mechanical Support: Principles and Practice, Glenn P. Gravlee, Davis, Richard 7. F, Alfred H. Stammers, Ungerleider, Ross M.
8. Manual of perioperative care in cardiac surgery, R.M.Bojar.

LIST OF FIGURES

1. https://www.geeksforgeeks.org/lung-volumes-and-capacities.
2. https://www.hamiltoncompany.com/process-analytics/dissolved-oxygen-knowledge/considerations-for- oxygen-measurement/ partial-and-absolute-pressure
3. Respiratory Physiology – Part 2 : WFSA - Resources.
4. https://resources.wfsahq.org/atotw/respiratory-physiology-part-2/
5. http://www5.zzu.edu.cn/__local/0/DB/69/1CEBD018 0B678808F07E75E0975_246AD76E_1F86C4.pdf?e=.pdf
6. https://www.dotmed.com/news/story/19389
7. https://www.ahajournals.org/doi/10.1161/CIRCULATIONAHA.108.830174
8. https://onih.pastperfectonline.com/webobject/F0BEA5C5-61B9-4CEA-9A59-809256575560 .
9. https://wellcomecollection.org/works/dkyepeaq
11. https://www.ahajournals.org/doi/10.1161/CIRCULATIONAHA.108.830174
12. https://www.ncbi.nlm.nih.gov/pmc/articles/PMC5683297/
13. https://www.annalsthoracicsurgery.org/article/S0003-4975(03)01820-4/fulltext
14. https://www.slideshare.net/Drvasanthi/oxygenators
15. https://m.indiamart.com/proddetail/adult-bubble-oxygenators-10742800455.html
16. https://terumo-asiapacific.com/cvs/product/capiox-fx-advance-oxygenators/ .
17. https://www.researchgate.net/figure/A-variable-Prime-Cobe-Membrane-Lung-and-B-Shiley-Plexus-35-Note-Courtesy-of-Sorin_fig6_304573983..
18. https://www.indiamart.com/proddetail/arterial-filter-adult-pead-infant-2572741112.html.
19. https://www.scanatron.com/en/performance/medical-technology/sechrist-gas-blenders-and-gas-tubes/.

20. https://sigmamotorinc.com/wpsigma/ .
21. https://americanhistory.si.edu/collections/search/object/nmah_998420
22. https://www.researchgate.net/figure/Centrifugal-Blood-Pump-A-plastic-cones-or-impeller-is-mounted-inside-the-conical_fig4_24283174https://www.researchgate.net/figure/Centrifugal-Blood-Pump-A-plastic-cones-or-impeller-is-mounted-inside-the-conical_fig4_24283174.
23. https://thoracickey.com/blood-pumps-circuitry-and-cannulation-techniques-in-cardiopulmonary-bypass/
24. https://thoracickey.com/blood-pumps-circuitry-and-cannulation-techniques-in-cardiopulmonary-bypass/
25. https://www.brainkart.com/article/Cardiopulmonary-Bypass_26978/.
26. https://aneskey.com/cardiopulmonary-bypass-equipment-circuits-and-pathophysiology-2/. .
27. https://www.uptodate.com/contents/management-of-cardiopulmonary-bypass/print.
28. https://www.indiamart.com/proddetail/cardiopulmonary-bypass-connectors-20763898891.html.
29. https://bioprocessintl.com/sponsored-content/ultrasonic-flow-and-bubble-sensors-made-from-piezocomposites-optimize-process-quality-in-single-use-bioprocessing-applications/.
30. https://www.researchgate.net/figure/Conventional-ultrafiltration-circuit-from-the-arterial-cannula-through-line-C-3-16_fig1_13083621.
31. https://perfusion.com/modified-ultrafiltration-during-cardiopulmonary-bypass/.
32. https://investor.masimo.com/news/news-details/2021/Study-Investigates-the-Effects-of-Ventilatory-Rescue-Therapies-on-the-Cerebral-Oxygenation-of-COVID-19-Patients-Using-Masimo-O3/default.aspx.
33. https://www.hamiltonhealthsciences.ca/share/perfusionist-lee-noble/.
34. https://www.livanova.com/cardiopulmonary/en-in/oxygenators/pediatrics.

INDEX

A

ABS or Acrylonitrile butadiene styrene, 48
acid citrate-phosphate-dextrose, 67
acid-base disorders, 120
ACT, 102
albumin, 70
Allen, 56
alveolar membrane, 15
Aminophylline, 115
Amplatz, 54
Andreasen and Watson, 58
anion gap, 121
Anticoagulation, 109
antithrombin interaction, 116
antithrombin, 113
anti-Xa levels, 111
apixaban, 113
aprotinin, 106
Argatroban, 113
arterial CO_2, 91
arterial-alveolar O_2 gradient, 121
arteriovenous shunting, 75
atmospheric gases, 17
atrial fibrillation (AF), 113
atropine, 115
autoclaving, 30
azygos flow principle, 58
Azygos flow principle, 67
azygos vein, 58

B

banked blood, 67
Barnard and Schrire, 105
Bigelow, 59
biofilm, 38
Bioline, 44
Biomedicus, 65
bispectral index (BIS), 90
Bivalirudin, 113
blood gas analyzer, 118
body mass index (BMI), 73
body surface area, or BSA, 68
Bretschneider, 82
bubble oxygenator, 32

C

Calcium Chloride, 116
capillary endothelium, 23
Capiox, 35
cardioplegia, 80
Cardioplegia, 81
cardiotomy, 81
Catecholamine
  infusions, 115
central venous
  pressure, 89
centrifugal pump, 63
Centrifugal pumps, 56
cerebral oximetry, 69
cerebroprotective, 106
cerebrospinal (CSF)
  drainage, 90
cerebrovascular accidents
  (CVA), 70
chatter, 124
citrate-phosphate-
  dextrose and
  adenosine, 67
classical method, 127
classical, 127
coarctation correction, 57
colloids, 69
complements, 82
connectors, 55
continuous cardiac output
  (CO), 91
controlled cross-
  circulation, 25
Conventional
  ultrafiltration
  (CUF), 86
Cooley-Beall, 32
Corticosteroids, 116
crystalloids, 69
Custodiol HTK, 83
custom packs, 49

D

Dale-Shuster, 28
D-dimer, 43
De-aeration, 70
De-airing, 67
deep hypothermic
  cerebral arrest
  (DHCA), 53
defoamation, 26
Del Nido
  solution, 83
delivery of oxygen
  (DO_2), 73
desferrioxamine, 106
DeWall, 25
Diabetic, 73
dialyser, 38
diatomaceous
  earth, 112
Dideco, 35

Diffusion, 15
Dilution, 67
Dodrill-GMR 'Michigan Heart', 63
Dubois formula, 98
Durant position, 126

E

$ECCO_2R$, 42
ECG, 89
ECMO, 42
edoxaban, 113
EEG, 106
endothelium, 15
ephedrine, 115
ETCO, 91
$ETCO_2$, 89
Ethyl Vinyl Acetate (EVA), 48
ethylcellulose, 38
exsanguination, 66
extracorporeal life support systems, 66
extracorporeal membrane oxygenation (ECMO), 65

F

factor Xa inhibitors, 113
fibrinogen, 43
Filters, 45, 79
Finger or piano key pumps, 56
Fleisch, 57
flow-meter, 66
fluorocarbons, 46
Forrest Dodrill, 57
fosphenytoin, 106
fraction of inspired oxygen (FiO_2), 95
functional residual capacity (FRC), 16

G

Gas blender, 46
General Motors, 58, 62
Gibbon, 24
gradient, 102
Griepp, 106
Gross, 57

H

Hagen–Poiseuille equation, 65
hard-shell polycarbonate, 35
Hematocrit, 67
hemodilution, 68
hemoglobin, 17
hemolysis, 40
hemotherm, 93
heparin, 42

heparin-induced thrombocytopenia (HIT-I and HIT-II), 112
hexadimethrine bromide (Polybrene), 114
hibernating animals, 103
Hollow Fiber, 39
hydrophilic membranes, 38
Hydrophobic isomers, 38
hyperoxic, 101
Hypokalemia, 121
Hypothermia, 59, 104
IBM, 57
IMO, 42

I

impellers, 64
in-line monitoring, 92
inspiratory capacity (IC), 16
integrated arterial line filtration (IALF) system, 46
internal diameter (ID), 80
interstitial fluid, 23
intra-aortic balloon pump (IABP), 94
Ionic balance, 68
IVOX, 42

J

Jostra Rotaflow, 65
Jules Verne, 27

K

kaolin, 112
Kay- Cross, 28
Kay, 27
Kerr, 82
Kirklin, 26
Kole chamber, 83
kymograph, 28

L

lactate, 74
Latex, 60
Le Gallois, 27
Levitronix, 65
lidocaine, 106
Lillehei, 25
Low prime volume, 68
Ludwig and Schmidt, 27
Luer lock, 55
lung, 15

M

magnesium, 106
magnetic levitation, 64, 66
manifold, 38
mannitol, 106

Melrose, 38
membrane oxygenators, 38
metabolic process, 23
Michael DeBakey, 57
micro-aggregates, 46
microemboli, 112
microplegia, 84
microporous polyolefin, 40
milieu interior, 118
mini-bypass, 84
minimally invasive cardiac surgery, 54
mitral commissurotomy, 57
modified ultrafiltration (MUF), 86
monitors, 88
MPAP = Mean pulmonary airway pressure, 19
Nafamostat mesilate, 113
nafamostat, 106
Near-infrared spectroscopy (NIRS), 69

N

nitric oxide, 101
Non-microporous membranes, 42
non-occlusive, 66
normovolemic hemodilution, 69
NPH (Neutral Protamine Hagedorn) insulin, 115
Nylon (polyamide), 48
nylon net, 38

O

optical fluorescence and reflectance-based systems, 92
oscilloscope, 89
oxygen combustion (VO_2), 73
Oxygen, 17
oxyhemoglobin, 18

P

Pacifico, 51
$PaCO_2$, 43, 74
PaO_2, 43
Partial pressure, 21
PCWP = Pulmonary capillary wedge pressure, 19
PDA interruption, 57
peristaltic pumps, 59
Phenylephrine, 115
phosphorylcholine, 42

Phosphorylcholine, 44
pH-stat, 96
Piston-driven pumps, 56
plasma, 70
poly-4 - methyl-1-pentene (PMP), 42
Polycarbonate, 48
Polyethylene (PE), 48
Polypropylene (PP), 48
polypropylene, 39
Polystan, 35
polytetrafluoroethylene (PTFE), 38
Polyurethane (PU), 48
Polyvinyl Chloride (PVC), 48
poly-vinyl-chloride (PVC), 31
Porter and Bradley, 56
priming volume, 68
pronto, 127
Protamine Sulfate Injection, 114
protamine, 111, 114
PTCA stenting, 113
pulmonary vascular resistance (PVR), 19
PULSATILITY, 85
pulse contour cardiac output - PCCO, 91
purge line, 79
$PvCO_2$, 74

R

reactive, 97
recombinant inactive antithrombin (rAT), 117
recombinant platelet factor P4 (Intravenous rPF4), 117
red blood cells, 18
reducers, 55
reserve capacities, 16
residual volume (RV), 16
Respiration, 18
respiratory quotient, 21
Retrograde autologous priming (RAP), 68
Revolution, 65
Rheopak, 44
Rheoparin, 44
r-Hirudin, 113
ripple mattress, 93
rivaroxaban, 113
Robert Hooke, 27
roller pump, 56
Roller pumps, 63

S

sandblasting, 51
Seldinger, 54
selectively permeable, 37
Sigma-motor pump, 62

silicone, 60
single-stage cannulae, 54
snuggers, 52
sodium bicarbonate, 120
solubility of gases, 21
somatosensory potential, 106
spectrophotometric, 92
Spictra, 35
spirometer, 28
SpO_2, 89
St. Thomas' solution, 82
stop-watch, 112
Strict asepsis, 68
superficial temporal artery, 88
superior vena cava (SVC), 107
Surface coating materials (SMA), 44
sweep, 101
Systemic Vascular Resistance (SVR), 77

T

Terumo, 35
Thermoregulation, 103
thrombocytopenia, 112
thromboxane A_2 receptor blockers, 106
tidal volume, 15
Tirofiban, 113
total lung capacity (TLC), 16
total lung volume/capacity, 15
transatrial, 54
transcatheter ventricular assist devices, 66
transcranial Doppler, 107
trans-septal venting, 82
Trendelenburg, 126
true silicone membranes, 39
Tullu, 94
Tumor necrosis factor (TNF), 82
two stage cannula, 54

U

ultrasonic bubble sensor, 92
unidirectional, 62

V

vascular resistances, 21
vasodilatation, 104
venous antegrade prime (VAP), 68
ventilation/perfusion (V/Q) ratio, 20

ventilation/perfusion (V/Q), 95
ventricular assist device (VAD), 65
ventricular assist device [VAD], 94
Vents, 77
Venturi, 125
vertical screen oxygenator, 30
vital capacity (VC), 16
Von Frey and Gruber, 28
Von Schroeder, 27

W

West zones, 20
William Mustard, 57

X

zero-balance ultrafiltration (ZBUF), 87
α-stat, 96

www.ingramcontent.com/pod-product-compliance
Ingram Content Group UK Ltd.
Pitfield, Milton Keynes, MK11 3LW, UK
UKHW022119230426
12048UKWH00010BA/604